THE WORLD OF MENTAL HEALTH

AN ESSENTIAL RESOURCE FOR FAMILIES, COUPLES, AND SINGLES

GABRIEL G. FELDMAR

WestBow
PRESS
A DIVISION OF THOMAS NELSON

WestBow Press books may be ordered through booksellers or by contacting:

WestBow Press
A Division of Thomas Nelson
1663 Liberty Drive
Bloomington, IN 47403
www.westbowpress.com
1-(866) 928-1240

ISBN: 978-1-4497-8784-4 (sc)
ISBN: 978-1-4497-8785-1 (hc)
ISBN: 978-1-4497-8783-7 (e)

Library of Congress Control Number: 2013904508

Printed in the United States of America

WestBow Press rev. date: 3/20/2013

SIGMUND FREUD (large image): Austrian physician/psychoanalyst (1856-1939)
CARL GUSTAV JUNG (standing): Swiss physician/psychoanalyst (1875-1961)
IVAN PETROVICH PAVLOV (sitting): Russian physician/physiologist (1849-1936)
OLD VIENNA (background): Illustration by Suzanne Feldmar, graphic artist
Cover page and interior illustrations were designed by Suzanne Feldmar

About this book...

The material in this book is helpful for readers who need information about the nature of a variety of common psychological and mental health topics. Included are areas related to child development, effective child rearing techniques, adolescent adjustment, adult relationships, mental illnesses in children and adults, description of mental health providers, diagnostic methods, types of medications and psychotherapy, psychiatric hospitalization, and the legal rights of mentally ill individuals.

DEDICATION

To my Parents, Katy, Suzanne, and Monique

ACKNOWLEDGMENT

I wish to thank my mother, Clara Feldmar, and my father, Tibor Feldmar, for encouraging me to write this book. Their continued support and practical ideas gave me the strength to accomplish this work. I am grateful to my colleagues, Marshall Silverstein, Ph.D., Dalit Matatyaho, Ph.D., Howard Sovronsky, L.C.S.W., and Seeth Vivek, M.D., for their most valuable suggestions related to this manuscript. I also appreciate the help of Alyssa Feldman in the preparation of the reference material related to this book.

My special thanks go to Suzanne Feldmar for her creative artistic efforts and illustrations related to this work.

TABLE OF CONTENTS

PREFACE

I have been working in the mental health field for over twenty-five years in a variety of clinical, research, educational settings and capacities. I have interacted with patients of all ages who had many different types of problems and disorders. Over the years of my practice I have made numerous observations and learned a great deal from the patients I treated. I also realized that there are certain fundamental facts, which must be addressed in order to achieve successful treatment outcomes and relapse preventive measures. These facts have to do with information and education about the nature of mental illness, the meaning of normal and abnormal behavior, the elements of interpersonal relationships, psychodevelopmental milestones, and general behavioral dynamics. Patients who possess some knowledge about these topics, and are open and psychologically minded, usually derive more benefit from mental health services than those who have no such understanding. Furthermore, information related to the nature of psychological, psychopharmacological, and substance abuse treatments are also very important for patients to know in order to maximize positive and long-lasting results from therapeutic interventions. It has come to my attention in the course of my work that most individuals who seek mental health services are quite uninformed about the nature of the services available to them.

The purpose of this book is to serve as a resource to better understand concepts related to mental health and mental illness. It is also my intent to educate the public about the nature of current psychological and psychiatric services. Information found in this book is based upon my clinical experience, and results of scientific studies conducted by qualified researchers. It is my hope that reading this material will result in improved appreciation for behavioral abnormalities, mental illnesses, treatment approaches, and the role of providers of mental health services. It is my belief that elimination of misconceptions in these areas will lead to the reduction of stigma related to mental illness, as well as a better understanding of when and where to look for psychological help. Treatment expectations will also become more realistic on the part of the "educated" consumer of mental health services.

This book is intended to be a reference manual for the general public, a guide, which will equip the reader with tools for the prevention of certain mental irregularities, improvement in the quality of psychological well being, and for conducting a more harmonious family and social life. This book will benefit not only people who are in need of mental health services. The information herein is designed to be beneficial for individuals and families regardless of their mental health status. Parents will be able to track the psychological development of their children, and adjust care-taking requirements accordingly. Appropriate parenting and behavior modifying skills will be learned to deal effectively with ever changing developmental and social needs. Early recognition of learning disabilities and related remediation options will be discussed. Issues related to family dynamics, and techniques needed to maintain a well-balanced marriage will be mentioned. Common, as well as less frequently encountered mental illnesses and substance abuse disorders will be explored. Personality factors related to social behavior will be addressed as well. Topics related to old age and care taking will also be examined. Lastly, in view of the fact that most people are unfamiliar with the law as it relates to psychiatry, I have added some important legal information.

I need to mention that the present volume is *not* a "quick-fix" manual for the solution to emergent behavioral problems. There already are an abundance of such manuals on bookstore shelves. In general they offer oversimplified "recipes" for the solution of complicated and deep-rooted problems. In most cases such methods are of minimal value. This book is a general reference tool for the understanding of basic psychological processes encountered in life. The appreciation of these processes will facilitate insight and a deeper familiarity with the self. Knowledge related to the psychological necessities for a well-adjusted style of life is important. Happiness often resides in our ability to maximize our potentials. Some psychologists call this process "self-actualization". Skillful management of daily stressors is also needed for securing optimal mental and physical health. Prompt attention to psychological problems in children, adolescents and adults are necessary to maximize treatment outcome. It is my vision that reading this book will result in a more fundamental understanding of our emotional, intellectual and social processes as we go through the span of life. This understanding will then result in improved adjustment, and a better quality of life. It is also my hope that the reader will have developed the required sensitivity to seek help when needed through the many avenues of available counseling and treatment options.

I organized this book according to related clusters of topic areas. The first three chapters address developmental concepts staring with conception through late adulthood. Basic physical, cognitive, emotional and social domains are described. Parent-child relationships are explored as well. Chapters four, five and six deal with mental health related issues such as stress management, categories of mental illnesses, psychological testing procedures and diagnostic methods used in psychiatry. Chapter seven introduces the various types of mental health providers, as well as the psychological and biological treatment approaches currently in use. Chapter eight, the final chapter, discusses the civil rights of individuals with mental illness. Every effort was made to avoid excessive technical language, and to expose the contents in an interesting albeit professional manner.

CHAPTER ONE:

Children and Adolescents

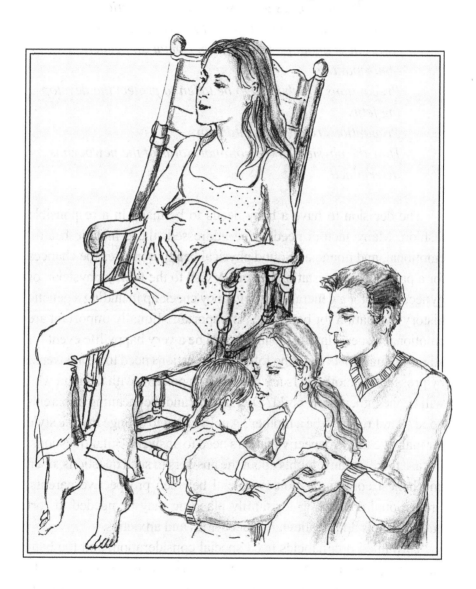

*"Maturity, one discovers, has everything to
do with the acceptance of 'not knowing'."*
MARK Z. DANIELEWSKI

SECTION 1.1:
CONCEPTION, PREGNANCY AND BIRTH

The following topics are discussed in this section:
How to make decisions related to having children
Awareness about possible chromosomal and genetic
abnormalities
Precautions which need to be taken to protect the develop-
ing fetus
Precautions related to childbirth
How the physical and emotional status of the newborn is
determined

The decision to have a baby needs to be made in a responsible fashion. Many factors need to be addressed; these include health, emotional, and financial. Sound physical health improves the chances for a problem free gestation period. A visit to the family physician or gynecologist for a general pre-pregnancy check up including a genetic history evaluation for both sexes is important. Equally important are emotional issues. Having a baby should be a very happy life event for all individuals involved. The following questions need to be answered by prospective mothers: Is my relationship positive with the man who will be the father of my child? Do I understand the meaning of parenthood? Am I ready to be a mother? Am I willing to change my life style for many years? Prospective fathers need to answer similar questions. In case there are any doubts about the answers to such questions, open and honest communication is crucial between prospective parents. Professional counseling for family planning may be needed to sort out dilemmas and to alleviate insecurities and anxieties.

Unwanted pregnancies need special consideration, and the benefit of responsible counseling may be very advantageous. How to find well-credentialed therapists will be discussed in later chapters. Visiting and talking to friends who already have children often helps in conceptualizing the realities surrounding family life and parenting. Financial and other practical considerations need to be figured out as

2

well. Does the family have sufficient income to support a child? If both parents will need to work, who will take care of the baby during working hours? Are nearby relatives willing to help with babysitting? Is there sufficient physical space at home to accommodate the expanding family? While these questions may sound elementary, thinking about them realistically may avert later panic.

Let us now examine some potential biological concerns. Chromosomal and genetic abnormalities are very common. Although approximately fifty percent of all human conceptions have abnormalities of this kind, fortunately many happen to be recessive (not physically expressed). Furthermore, normal genes of one parent often counteract the effects of the defects introduced by the other parent. Genotypic abnormalities, on the other hand, have been detected in about three to four percent of newborns (Ward, 1994). In cases of concern, prospective parents are advised to consult pediatricians about options for genetic counseling. The following is a list of common genetic conditions and diseases. A brief description and associated prognosis is also listed:

Phenylketonuria: Brain development is inhibited by lack of an enzyme. A restricted diet can prevent severe mental retardation.

Down syndrome: Chromosomal abnormality resulting in various levels of mental retardation. Special education and/or institutionalization is needed to maximize functional potentials. Many children and adults with Down syndrome can function at high levels and achieve considerable independence.

Turner syndrome: Secondary sex characteristics fail to develop in females. Treatment is questionable.

Cystic fibrosis: The lungs and digestive tract become obstructed by mucus. This enzymatic abnormality results in a very short life span, often not reaching adulthood. .

Hemophilia:	Abnormality in the blood clotting mechanism may result in dangerous internal bleeding. Frequent transfusions may be needed to stabilize the condition.
Sickle cell anemia:	Severe anemia and circulatory problems are caused by abnormal red blood cells. While the condition is disabling, it is treatable with medication.
Klinefelter syndrome:	Secondary sex characteristics fail to develop in males. Treatment is often not successful.
Thalassemia:	Abnormal red blood cells, resulting in enlarged liver and spleen. Poor motivation, flat affect. Condition may be fatal. Blood transfusions may be effective.
Neurofibromatosis:	Benign tumors on peripheral and optic nerves. Learning disabilities. Surgery may be of help.
Tay-Sachs disease:	Toxins build up in brain tissue as a result of a lack of an enzyme. Early death in childhood as a result of neurological degeneration (Cole et al, 2005; Jorde et al., 1999; Rimoin et al., 1997; Simpson & Golbus, 1993.)

Prenatal development is usually divided into three parts. The *germinal period* begins at the time of conception when the male and female germ cells are joined. This period ends when the developing organism attaches itself to the wall of the uterus. This process takes about ten days. The *embryonic period* takes about eight weeks. During this period the major organs begin to develop, and have a primitive shape. The *fetal period* extends until childbirth. During this period the major organs develop, and the baby is prepared to be able to survive without physiological maternal support (Shaffer, 2002). Prospective mothers need to be cognizant of a variety of conditions that affect the developing fetus. These conditions include general health, various environmental factors, nutrition, her emotional state, stress, and her attitude toward having a baby. Research results tell us that unwanted babies weigh less and need more medical support than babies whose mothers are happy with their pregnancy.

Excessive stress can also be harmful. Elevated levels of *cortisol* and *adrenaline* (stress hormones), which cross the placenta, can have long lasting negative emotional effects on children (Relier, 2001). Low birth weight, premature delivery, elevated motor activity and increased aggression have been observed in these children (Lobel, 1994; Susman et.al. 2001). Essential vitamins and minerals and a well balanced diet of 2000 to 2800 calories are recommended (Christian, 2002). In addition, health care providers often advise increased intake of folic acid (vitamin B), iron and calcium. Including small amounts of zinc and magnesium to the mother's diet can reduce birth complications (Friedman & Polifka, 1996). According to some studies deficient maternal nutrition can lead to miscarriage, low birth weight, premature birth, and a greater risk for the development of stroke, and heart disease later in life (Godfrey & Barker, 2000; Mora & Nestel, 2000).

There are many *teratogens* (environmental toxic agents), which may cause serious damage to the developing embryo and fetus. Severe structural and physiological birth defects are associated with a variety toxic substances. Abnormal development of internal organs and external body parts are frequently seen. Such damages are irreversible and are often fatal. Susceptibility to teratogenic agents partially depends on genetic vulnerability to such sources. The mother's physiological state is also a factor. Hormonal balance, maternal nutrition, and age are relevant factors as well. Mothers who are less than twenty and older than forty years old pose most risk to the developing baby. Pollution, ingestion of certain drugs, infection and exposure to radiation are the most common sources for birth defects.

Pollution in industrialized societies is a great concern. Much is said about this problem in the media, and in political circles, but unfortunately too little is being done to eliminate this concern. Herbicides, pesticides, food additives, oil spills in our waterways, industrial waste products such as mercury, and air pollution from petrochemical plants constitute ongoing environmental hazards.

Substance abuse, including alcohol and tobacco is a serious social problem in the United States. Both alcohol and tobacco, including exposure to second-hand cigarette smoke, may harm the developing fetus. Abstinence during pregnancy is therefore strongly advised. Nearly half of the adult population in our country has used an illicit drug at some point in their lives. Approximately one in ten adults in our country engage in substance abuse at some point during their span of life. Many pregnant women take non-prescription pain relievers, and sleep medication. Some also take pills to counteract nausea. While most of these medications are harmless, we have no conclusive research evidence about teratogenic (toxic effect which cause birth defects) effects of all over-the-counter medications; therefore minimal or no use is the safest approach. Many classes of prescription medications have been found to cause abnormalities in the developing fetus. These include artificial hormones, some antipsychotic medications (e.g. Thorazine), anxiolytic medications (e.g. Valium), many antibiotics, anticonvulsants, and anticoagulants (Chavkin, 1995). The following is a list of commonly used illicit drugs and their teratogenic effects:

Heroin: This drug is a derivative of opium, and is highly addictive. It can be smoked, inhaled as a powder, or injected under the skin or directly into the bloodstream. It has pain-relieving and sleep-inducing properties. Addicted mothers give birth to babies who are addicted as well. Very often these babies are born prematurely, and are underweight. They may be at risk to develop respiratory illnesses (Kaltenbach et. al., 1998). They need to be weaned off heroin under careful medical supervision in order to avoid life threatening withdrawal reactions.

Methadone: Methadone hydrochloride is a synthetic narcotic which under medical supervision is used to reduce the cravings for heroin. It is available in some drug rehabilitation programs. Babies whose mothers use this drug are born addicted. Upon birth they need to be given methadone in order to avoid often fatal sudden withdrawal effects. These babies often have tremors, are irritable, and have sleep disturbances.

Cocaine: Cocaine is a natural stimulant found in the leaves of the coca plant. The hardened form of cocaine is called "crack". Cocaine can be sniffed, smoked or injected (Nevid, 2013). In some South American countries tea is brewed from coca leaves, and ingested as a beverage. Cocaine users enjoy a feeling of euphoria. Addicted mothers are at risk for depression, psychosis, anxiety, damage to the heart and circulatory system, respiratory arrest and strokes. (Cunningham et al., 2001). Overdose can be fatal. The effects on baby include irritability, poor coordination, learning disabilities and hyper-reactivity to environmental stimulation. (Bendersky & Lewis, 1998). Some residual symptoms may affect cognitive and emotional development for years.

Marijuana: Marijuana is derived from the leaves and flowering tops of the plant Cannabis sativa (Butcher, et al., 2007). It is considered to be a mild hallucinogen. Smokers of this drug report subjective feelings of relaxation and euphoria. At higher doses it can produce perceptual distortions The effects on the baby is often associated with premature birth and low birth weight.

We often do not think of alcohol as a "drug". The reasons behind excessive alcohol use however, is very similar to those which lead people to drug abuse. Mind altering properties of alcohol, which appeal to the user, include a temporary pleasant mood, elevated self-esteem and an escape from the stressful effects of reality. Alcohol addiction may result upon repeated drinking. Chronic alcoholism often has irreversible and fatal physical effects, such as *cirrhosis of the liver* (irreversible scarring of liver tissue). *Alcohol amnestic disorder* (alcohol-related psychosis) is another severe side effect, the main symptom of which is profound memory loss especially for recent events. The teratogenic (abnormal malformations) effects of alcohol include serious birth defects such as congenital heart disease, abnormally small head with facial deformities. Brain damage and joint and eye abnormalities also occur. *Fetal alcohol syndrome*, which includes these anomalies, usually results in retarded physical and mental development. It is essential therefore for pregnant women to refrain from the ingestion of alcohol (Calhoun & Warren, 2007). Tobacco, as mentioned above, may also have serious harmful effects on the fetus. These include stillbirth, miscarriages, and neonatal death (Chan, Keane & Robinson, 2001). Smoking during pregnancy may also lead to disruptive behavior in children (Wakschlag et al., 2006). Lower birth weight results from the adverse effects of nicotine on placental growth (Chertok, et al., 2011). As a result from abnormal growth of the placenta the fetus does not receive sufficient nutrients and oxygen. As stated above, prospective mothers are strongly advised to stop smoking, and to avoid smoky environments.

Excessive caffeine consumption has been linked to increased probability for miscarriage and low birth weight (CARE Study Group, 2008). Consequently, only limited or no intake of coffee, tea, and cola drinks are recommended for pregnant women.

In addition to drugs and other ingestible substances there are other dangers to the embryo, fetus and the newborn, which need to be kept in mind. Pregnant women who suffer from Rubella, or German measles may give birth to babies with mental retardation, congenital heart disease, cataracts and deafness (Bale, 2002). Prospective mothers should receive vaccinations at least six months prior to conception. Medical consultation is recommended.

The following are some additional maternal diseases and conditions, which may affect prenatal development: Genital herpes, Gonorrhea, Syphilis, Chicken pox, Cytomegalovirus, Diabetes, Hepatitis, Hypertension, Influenza, Mumps, Toxemia, and Toxoplasmosis (Jones, Lopez, & Wilson, 2003; Kliegman et al., 2008; Moore & Persaud, 1993; Stevenson, 1977). Babies born to mothers with *Acquired Immunodeficiency Syndrome (AIDS)* are at risk for developing the disease. The virus may be transmitted through the placental barrier. Also, at the time of delivery the baby may become exposed to the mother's infected blood (Cole, Cole, & Lightfoot, 2005). The *human immunodeficiency virus (HIV)* is very aggressive and produces devastating damage to infants. This includes serious brain damage, respiratory illnesses, diarrhea, and death (Devi et. al., 2009). Preconception exposure to HIV/AIDS needs to be determined in order to receive proper medical advice and care prior and during pregnancy. Medications are currently available to reduce the baby's chances of infection. *Rh incompatibility* (a characteristic of red blood cells) also needs to be discussed with the treating physician in order to prevent birth defects in future pregnancies (Shaffer, 2002). Exposure to radiation must be minimized during pregnancy in order to avoid serious malformations to the developing fetus (Vorhees & Mollnow, 1987). Pregnant women must alert their physicians and dentists.

Childbirth is a psychologically happy event, but physically painful. *Analgesics* (pain killers) and *sedatives* (tranquilizers) are often prescribed to control pain. Unfortunately these medications have undesirable effects on the newborn. Symptoms include irritability, poor muscle tone, reduced attention, and less vigorous sucking responses (Caton et al., 2002). Many pregnant women elect alternative modes of pain control, such as relaxation and breathing exercises. Most hospitals offer educational classes to teach women these self-help skills. Medical interventions such as inducing labor and cesarean section are needed when the mother's life is in danger or when the baby is in distress during delivery. Sometimes these procedures are recommended unnecessarily and need to be discussed carefully with obstetricians.

The *Apgar Scale* is often used in delivery rooms to determine the physical condition of the newborn. Heart rate, respiratory effort, muscle tone, reflex responsivity, and color are examined (Apgar, 1953). The *Brazelton Neonatal Assessment Scale* is used to assess the neurological condition of babies who may be at risk for developmental problems. This test measures muscle tone, reflexes, motor capacities, capacity for responding to environmental stimulation, and attention (Brazelton & Nugent, 1995). Infants who are premature (born before the 37th week of gestational period) and of low birth weight (under 5.5 lbs.) are at risk for poor coordination, attentional problems, and intellectual slowing. These babies require additional medical and psychological care in order to avoid future disabilities.

Prior to birth parents frequently have imaginations and expectations related to the forthcoming baby's appearance and abilities. Upon the arrival of the baby some of these expectations may or may not be realized. The total and unconditional acceptance of the newborn by parents cannot be overstated. The development of a close bond between parents and baby is crucial for optimal physical and psychological development. Infants are totally dependent on the continuous care of parents. Research results in developmental psychology indicate that the parent-child relationship is determined by a number of factors. These include the personality, education, and upbringing of the parents, socioeconomic conditions of the family, the temperament and behavior of the baby, the health condition and physical appearance of the baby. Mothers find it difficult to care for infants with physical birth defects or behavioral abnormalities. Timely consultation with pediatricians and child psychologists is important. Attractive babies often get more parental attention than less attractive ones. Friendly and smiling babies also enjoy more parental interaction. These findings will be explored further in later chapters.

SECTION 1.2:
PHYSICAL DEVELOPMENT OF THE INFANT

The following topics are discussed in this section:
The neurological development of the infant, including essential reflexes
The relationship between biological and psychological development
The chronology of sensory and motor development

The brain is the organ of behavior. Both primitive and socialized behaviors are determined by brain development. Sensory-motor functions, emotional and social experiences, and intellectual functioning are included. Even before they are born, the *central nervous system* (brain and spinal cord) of fetuses is rather well developed. The fetus is able to recognize and respond to certain sounds, and make spontaneous movements. At the time of birth, the brain contains most of the cells it will need for the continuity of life. The complexity of these cells, called *neurons* will increase dramatically in the process of growth. The human brain, especially the cerebral cortex (the part of the brain involved in cognitive functions), contains more than 100 billion nerve cells. This is a major distinguishing factor between our species (homo sapiens) and other animals.

Information is transmitted between neurons in the form of small electrical impulses. Transmission to muscle and gland cells is also possible. Neurons have unique structural characteristics, which set them apart from other body cells. It is important to become familiar with the structure and function of neurons to fully appreciate the normal or abnormal physical and psychological development of children. Conditions such as hyperactivity and learning disabilities are also related to neuronal activities. Most serious mental illnesses have major biological foundations involving the electrical and biochemical properties of neurons.

The mechanism of action of psychoactive medications (medications which affect mental processes and behavior) also takes place at the level of the neuron. The basic structure of neurons includes a main protruding branch called the *axon*. The branches, which arise at the surface of the nerve cell, are called *dendrites*. The *synapse* is a tiny gap between the axon of one cell and the dendrite of the neighboring adjoining cell. When an electrical impulse propagated along the axon arrives at the synapse, the tiny receptacles at the axon terminals secrete a biochemical substance into the synapse. This substance is called a *neurotransmitter*. The neurotransmitter then carries the impulse across the synapse to the neighboring receiving neuron. One axon may be in contact with only a few receiving neurons, or with very many others. The complexity of brain activity is in many ways the function of an infinite variety of neuronal networks. These neuronal networks regulate many psychological events. Perception, memory, intellectual and emotional processes are all involved. *Myelin* is another important part of the neuron. This is a fatty substance, which insulates axons. The insulation results in a more rapid transmission of nerve impulses. Disturbance in myelination results in serious neurological disorders such as multiple sclerosis.

The brain has the capacity to undergo structural changes in response to environmental experience and learning. New synaptic connections are formed, and neurochemical changes take place as we go through life and gain more experience. Nonfunctional synapses selectively die off. There is an ongoing dynamic correlation in the brain between psychological and physiological processes. The developmental morphology and organization of the brain is very complex, and is beyond the intended scope of this volume. Some important brain structures and functions however will be discussed. The *cerebral cortex* is the brain's outermost layer. It is here that most cognitive processes take place. Psychological and physical developmental milestones are often related to the biological status of the cerebral cortex.

It is important to realize that the brain has many roles other than just "thinking". Some important brain involvement includes heartbeat, respiration, sleeping and arousal and physical movement and coordination. Sensory stimulation and the opportunity for physical activity are important for optimal and timely development during infancy. Overstimulation however is not advised. Sensitivity on the part of parents regarding the developmental *readiness* of infants is crucial. Stereotyped reflex activity in neonates is indicative of myelination of motor neurons. Continued myelination of the motor pathways in the brain is necessary for the normal development of sensorimotor capabilities. The process of myelination does not end in infancy. According to some researchers, this process continues into adolescence. Development of neurons required for the sense of hearing begins about the sixth month of pregnancy, and continues until about the age of four years. In infancy there is a rapid improvement in sensitivity to sound. Newborns are able to preferentially differentiate human voice from other kinds of sounds in the environment. Neuronal development necessary for vision begins toward the end of the gestation period, and lasts until about six months of age. Physiological readiness for color vision is almost completed at the time of birth. Visual acuity is poor in early infancy, but by seven or eight months of age acuity is greatly improved. Visual scanning develops very early in life. Pattern and object perception develops early as well. Babies less than two days old are able to distinguish among visual forms (Fantz, 1961). The perception of faces also develops early in life. Very soon following birth newborns are able to recognize their mother's face (Bushnell, 2001).

Both taste and smell are rather well developed at birth (Berk, 2013). This appears to be an important "self preservation" skill to protect babies from ingesting aversive and potentially hazardous substances. Furthermore, preference for sweet-tasting substances facilitates babies' desire to ingest nutritious liquids. By the second year of life myelination of the nerves associated with muscles is mostly completed. This is very needed for proper motor development. These nerves also facilitate coordination of movement and changes in posture. Motor development takes place in an orderly fashion. Control of the head and upper torso precedes control of arms. Control of trunk and shoulders precedes use of hands and fingers. (Rathus, 2006) Neonates are able to move their heads slightly to the side. By about two months, they can also lift their chests while lying on their stomachs. They can also hold their heads quite well by about three to six months. Because musculature is still weak at this age, careful handling of babies is necessary to prevent neck injuries. Lifting of infants should be accomplished gently, avoiding sudden and jerky movements.

Hand control is an exciting milestone. At first, grasping is reflexive. By the age of three to four months voluntary grasping develops. By the age of four to six months infants can transfer objects back and forth between hands. Use of the thumb does not take place until about nine to twelve months. About this time infants can also adjust their hands in anticipation of grasping moving objects (Claxton, Keen, & McCarthy, 2003). Between fifteen and twenty-four months, the further development of visual coordination allows infants to stack blocks (Wenworth, Benson, & Haith, 2000). By about two years of age they can also copy horizontal and vertical lines. Environmental opportunities combined with parental stimulation have a positive effect on these developmental milestones. Locomotion also evolves in a sequential manner. While there are some individual variations, the following motor developmental milestones are known: (Rathus, 2008)

24-28 weeks   Sitting up
32-36 weeks   Crawling
36-40 weeks   Kneeling
40-44 weeks   Creeping
44-52 weeks   Standing
52-64 weeks   Starting to walk
64-76 weeks   Full walking

The ability to move around enables infants to further explore their environment, and experience new social play activities and learning opportunities.

At the time of birth babies are equipped with some basic *sensory capacities*. These include hearing, vision, smell, taste, touch, temperature, and position. They show a preference for attending to their native language; they have blurred vision, but by two months of age they have color vision; they can differentiate between odors and tastes; they are responsive to touch, changes in temperature, and body position (Cole, 2005). A number of *reflexes* must be present at birth for normal neurological development to take place. The following is a list of essential reflexes and their description: (Feldman, 2012)

Babinski: When the bottom of the baby's foot is stroked, the toes fan out and then curl.

Crawling: When the baby is placed on his stomach and pressure is applied to the soles of his feet, his arms and legs move rhythmically.

Eyeblink: Rapid closing of eyes.

Grasping: When a finger or some other object is pressed against the baby's palm, her fingers close around it.

Moro: If the baby is allowed to drop unexpectedly while being held or if there is a loud noise, she will throw her arms outward, while arching her back and then bring her arms together as if grasping something.

Rooting: The baby turns his head and opens his mouth when he is touched on the cheek.

Stepping: When the baby is held upright over a flat surface, he makes rhythmic leg movements.

Sucking: The baby sucks when something is put into her mouth.

Startle: moving the arms, back and fingers response to sudden noise.

Gag: reflex to clear the throat.

By six to eight months of age infants will have relatively well developed *depth perception.* This ability protects them from injuries such as falling off a cliff, as they are crawling. *Perceptual constancies (size and shape)* also develop in early infancy. This ability allows infants to perceive objects as the same even though sensations produced by them may differ (Rathus, 2008.) For example a table has the shape of a rectangle no matter how it is moved or tilted.

Intermodal perception develops very early as well. It is the ability to use one sensory modality to identify a stimulus or pattern of stimuli that is already familiar through another modality. For example the ability to recognize a feeding bottle, with which the infant has visual familiarity, by touching it (Gibson & Walker, 1984).

SECTION 1.3:
COGNITIVE DEVELOPMENT OF THE INFANT

The following topics are discussed in this section:
Major theories of cognitive and language development
Stages of perceptual development
Development of learning and memory
Tests used to measure cognitive development

The meaning of cognitive development includes perception and mental representation of the physical and social environment, which surrounds the infant. The research and theories of the famous Swiss biologist Jean Piaget contributed much to our understanding of children's thought processes. According to Piaget all normally developing children go through four distinct *stages* of cognitive development (*Sensorimotor, Preoperational, Concrete Operational and Formal Operational*). In the course of the sensorimotor stage (birth to two years of age) infants use mental structures that are involved in the acquisition or organization of knowledge. Piaget named these structures *schemes*. He further posited that through the process of *assimilation* infants incorporate new events or knowledge into existing schemes. For example the scheme "cars" would allow for the incorporation of many types of cars into this mental structure. However seeing an airplane will require the development of a new conceptual category or the modification of an already existing category or scheme. This cognitive process is called *accommodation*. In normally developing children, these processes occur by two years of age. These cognitive developments take place via sensory (e.g. seeing or hearing) and motor (e.g. moving fingers and hands) activity, hence the term "sensorimotor". During this time span infants begin to shift focus from their own bodies to events and objects in the external environment. Intentional or goal directed behavior also begins to emerge.

Learning by imitation of unfamiliar actions as well as trial and error problem solving attempts are also evident. The understanding of *object permanence* during the first two years of age is very

17

important. This ability allows the infant to recognize that objects continue to exist even when they are out of sight. For example, the infant understands that her mother will continue to exist event when she leaves the bedroom and goes to the kitchen. The infant, therefore, will "expect" her return. The proper development of *working (short-term) memory* and *reasoning ability* are necessary in order for the infant to appreciate that "out of sight" does not necessarily mean "permanent cessation of existence" (Aguilar & Baillargeon, 2002).

Cognitive development incorporates several *information processing* skills. The ability to memorize and imitate arms infants with tools, which are needed for the processing of information. *Memory* is usually understood as having three components: *encoding (input), storage and retrieval.* Between two and six months of age, and then again around the twelfth month there is a dramatic improvement in memory (Pelphrey, et al., 2004). Biological brain development, and the opportunity and encouragement to learn are important determinants in this process. *Imitation* facilitates much of human learning. Shortly after birth infants have been seen to imitate certain limited aspects of adult behavior. Some of this behavior may be reflexive, and may facilitate caregiver-infant bonding (Meltzoff & Prinz, 2002). Many studies indicate that by six months of age imitation is voluntary rather than reflexive.

Lots of individual differences exist in the process of cognitive development. When significant developmental delay is suspected, an evaluation by a child psychologist is recommended. The *Bayley Scales of Infant Development* is a well-known instrument used for the measurement of infant intelligence. This test addresses mental, motor, and behavioral functions. The mental scale assesses memory, learning, sensory-perceptual abilities, problem solving, abstraction, mathematical concept formation, and verbal communication. The motor scale assesses gross motor skills, such as standing, walking, and climbing, and fine motor skills, such as hand and finger manipulations, as well as postural imitation. A behavioral rating scale based on examiner observation is also part of this test; arousal, attention span, emotional regulation, goal directedness, persistence, and aspects of social development are reported (Aiken & Groth-Marnat, 2006). Early detection of sensory and neurological problems is important as well. Two popular instruments for this purpose are the *Brazelton Neonatal Behavioral Assessment Scale* (as described earlier) and the *Denver Developmental Screening Test* (Aiken & Groth-Marnat, 2006). Abnormalities in any of these tests need to be taken seriously. Pediatricians, child psychologists and developmental rehabilitation specialists need to be consulted regarding the possible need for early intervention plans. Parents are often "obsessed" with trying to improve their infants' cognitive prowess. They often find themselves forever searching for "miracle products" in a variety of toy stores. There is really no need for such a search. Frequent communication with eye contact, playing, reading stories, involvement in routine activities, such as shopping in malls and supermarkets, allowing social contact with peers, and interesting excursions (e.g. zoos, interactive museums, circuses) provide sufficient learning opportunities for infants.

Language development takes place in a stepwise sequence. Language is a symbolic manner of communication in which events and objects are represented by words. In the beginning infants express themselves in *prelinguistic* vocalizations. Cooing, babbling and crying represent this type of communication. Between the ages of ten and fourteen months (sometimes as late as eighteen months) the infant begins to utter the first word. Parents are always delighted to witness this development. These first words are brief, ordinarily consisting of no more than two syllables. At this stage vocabulary development is slow for the next three to four months. Around sixteen to twenty-four months of age vocabulary develops more rapidly (Gleitman & Landau, 1994). Most new words learned are nouns. In general, through the preschool years children acquire an average of nine new words per day (Hoff, 2006). *Telegraphic speech* (brief expressions that have the meanings of sentences) begins to develop between eighteen and twenty-four months of age. Over the next several months telegraphic speech gradually declines, as full sentences begin to be used (Brown & Fraser, 1963).

Psychologists and psycholinguists proposed several theories of language development. Burrhus Frederic Skinner, the famous American behavioral psychologist, suggested that *reinforcement* has a major role in language development. He claimed that as parents *shape* their infants' utterances by consistent rewards, such as smiling and expressing approval, infants *learn* to differentiate between correct and incorrect pronunciation and word usage. Hence consistent reinforcing of proper imitation and systematically ignoring erroneous utterances promotes the development of vocabulary, grammar and *syntax* (the rules in a language for placing words in proper order to form sentences). Psycholinguist Noam Chomsky theorized that infants possess an innate tendency to acquire language. Evidence for this inborn tendency comes from studies of deaf and foreign-born children. Regular early production of sounds occurs even in deaf children. Furthermore, the development of language takes place in an organized, regular and predictable order regardless of the type of language the child is learning (Bloom, 1998). Most developmentalists agree that language acquisition, as are most other psychological processes, is a function of both biological and environmental influences. Neuropsychological and neuroradiological evidence indicates that the brain locations most involved in the production and comprehension of language are *Broca's and Wernicke's areas*, named after the scientists who discovered them. These areas are located on the left side of the brain.

SECTION 1.4:
SOCIAL AND EMOTIONAL DEVELOPMENT IN INFANCY

The following topics are discussed in this section:
The development of healthy and unhealthy attachment
Causes for emotional security and insecurity
Parenting techniques which optimize normal emotional
development
The effects of child abuse
Current knowledge related to autism
How to identify quality day care for infants
Chronology of emotional development
Major theories of personality development
Temperamental characteristics of infants
Suggestions for parents who have children with "difficult"
personalities

We often talk about *attachment*. In everyday parlance this means affection or love. Much research has been done on the nature of attachment. Child psychologist Mary Ainsworth is known for her work in this area. She defined "attachment" as an emotional tie formed between two organisms (animals or persons). Attachment is an enduring form of behavior, and keeps organisms together; it is essential for the survival of infants. Attachment development is most critical in the first year of life. Babies are born with certain capacities, such as smiling, clinging and crying, which promote the establishment of attachment between baby and caregiver (Ainsworth & Bowlby, 1991). *Separation anxiety* sets in when babies feel that contacts with primary caregivers are weakened.

Various *patterns of attachment* exist; some are healthy, others are detrimental to normal emotional development. Some forms of attachment are *secure*; others are *insecure*. Securely attached infants exhibit mild forms of protestations upon their mother's temporary departure, and visibly seek interaction upon her return. They also readily accept maternal comforting. Babies who show *avoidant*

21

attachment are least distressed by theirs mothers' temporary departure. They ignore their mothers upon reunion. Infants who show *ambivalent/resistant attachment* are very emotional; they show severe signs of distress when their mothers leave, and show ambivalence upon their return. They alternately cling to and push away their mothers. Insecure attachment is detrimental to mental health later in life. Securely attached infants are happier, and feel more comfortable with both familiar and unfamiliar adults. They tend to be more cooperative with their parents, and relate more sociably with peers. They usually behave more comfortably in school than children who are insecurely attached (Belsky, 2006). Securely attached children feel safer in unfamiliar environments, and more readily initiate contact with unfamiliar people. They also have longer attention spans and are less impulsive than insecurely attached infants (Englund et al., 2000). Insecure attachment may result in future psychological disorders at adolescence and adulthood.

How is attachment established? The quality of care infants receive has a lot to do with healthy attachment. Parental affection, availability, cooperation, attentiveness, consistency and predictability in their caregiving are important factors. When the quality of home life deteriorates for reasons such as frequent hostility between parents, separation and divorce or debilitating illness of parents, the nature of attachment will almost always suffer. When one or both parents are mentally ill, addicted to alcohol or drugs, or are abusive to their children, insecure attachment is often to be expected. Insecure attachment is also often seen in economically disadvantaged and broken families. Parent-child interaction is a two-way street. While parents' behavior and attitudes affect children, the converse is true as well. Baby's temperament, for example, is associated with security. Very active and irritable babies often develop insecure attachment; so do babies who frequently display negative emotions. Often such infants do not get sufficient and timely attention from their parents, because they are considered to be "difficult" children. Parents often find it hard to be emotionally close to babies with this type of temperament (Morrell & Steele, 2003).

Studies related to fathers' involvement in childrearing have indicated that differences exist between father-child interactions and mother-child interactions in the United States. In general fathers spend little time on tasks involving basic child-care. They preferentially engage themselves with play activities, at times physical rough-and-tumble play. Mothers on the other hand are very much involved with essential and daily child-care needs such as changing diapers, washing and feeding their babies. Infants' attachment to their parents is determined by the amount of "quality time" they spend with them. Frequent and affectionate interactions result in strong bonding. Most infants under stress, such as pain or fear, will look for their mothers for help and protection. This happens because mothers in general are more available, more responsive physically and emotionally, and are more involved with "life sustaining" needs of infants.

Social scientists and developmental psychologists have extensively explored the effects of life in some orphanages on the mechanism of attachment. The effects of negligent and abusing parenting have also been studied. Social deprivation and the absence of opportunity for attachment have severe negative effects on development. Impairment in emotional, social, intellectual, and physical development can be expected in institutionalized children who receive little or no social stimulation. Children in such predicaments frequently become withdrawn, despondent, and depressed (Fischer et al., 1997). Delays in language development, and self-stimulation in the form of rocking back and forth are often seen. Fortunately infants have the capacity to recover from the effects of social deprivation. They often regain normal intellectual, social and emotional functioning over time, as their environment and the quality of their caretaking improves (Clark & Hanisee, 1982).

Abuse by parents or caregivers leads to devastating psychological consequences as well. According to a recent survey conducted by the U.S. Department of Health and Human Services, nearly three million American children are neglected or abused psychologically, physically, or sexually each year by their parents or caregivers (U.S Department of Health and Human Services, 2004). It is suspected that this number is much larger though, because many abuse and neglect cases go unreported. Abuse frequently results in serious injuries requiring medical care and hospitalization. Thousands of children die as a consequence. Boys are more often than girls the targets of harsh treatment.

Sexual abuse of girls is very prevalent too. Fewer cases are seen with boys. Frequent headaches, stomachaches, and bedwetting occur in abused children. Naturally, these children are less securely attached to their parents, and often manifest psychological disorders. Their social behavior is marked by emotional constriction, less intimacy with peers, increased aggression, anger and noncompliance with behavioral guidelines set by adults (Joshi et.al., 2006; Straus & Gelles, 1990). The self-esteem of abused children is low. As a consequence of cognitive impairments their school performance is below average. They are often emotionally blunt and are hesitant approaching unfamiliar adults. Abuse in infancy has long lasting developmental effects. As these children reach adolescence, they will be at greater risk for a variety of delinquent behaviors and substance abuse (Eckenrode et al., 1993). In adulthood many of these children will have difficulties establishing romantic relationships. They will behave aggressively toward their intimate partners, resulting in separation or divorce.

What causes child abuse? There are several contributory factors to parental abuse. Stressful family life (e.g. poverty, infidelity), parental exposure to abuse, poorly developed coping mechanisms, ineffective parenting and problem-solving skills, alcoholism and substance abuse. Parents' lack of familiarity with developmental milestones, and consequent unrealistic expectations from their children may also result in abuse (Craig & Sprang, 2007; Kaufman & Zigler, 1992). When such expectations are not met, children may receive harsh punishment. Certainly major disruptions in family life, such as loss of income, legal problems, incarceration, severe physical or mental illness, separation, and divorce may also lead to abusive behavior, because parents lose patience and become easily annoyed by their children's crying and demands. Excessively active and poorly behaved children who are not responsive to parental guidance are usually more at risk for abuse, because they require more time and attention. While it is true that many abusive parents have been the victims of child abuse themselves, it is also true that most mothers and fathers, who were abused as children, do not abuse their own children (Straus & McCord, 1998). In fact many of them turn out to be caring and attentive average parents. Research has shown that child abuse often runs in families. In the course of psychological development parents serve as role models for their children.

Years of exposure to violence leads children to believe that screaming, hitting, throwing objects, and punching holes in walls are the accepted ways of dealing with stress and expressing anger. Eventually family violence becomes to be accepted as the "norm". These children will not have the opportunity to learn more socially adaptive behaviors of stress reduction, such as verbal expression of feelings, humor, breathing exercises or reasoning (Straus, 1995).

What kind of measures can be taken in the face of child abuse? Many states require anyone, but especially health care professionals such as nurses, psychologists and physicians to report any suspicion of child abuse to authorities. Both local and federal social agencies have funded parent-education classes. Some programs provide for home visitors such as social workers to help prospective and new parents with the acquisition of proper parenting skills, caregiving, and the general management of their families. Child abuse hotlines are available for parents who tend to be aggressive with their children. These services help callers manage their emotions in socially acceptable ways.

As concerned citizens, what can we do when we suspect cases of child sexual abuse? Foremost, we need to realize that sexually abused children are often hurt, feel shameful and guilty. Our approach to them needs to be gentle, gradual, calm and reassuring. The American Psychological Association suggests the following guidelines:

- Provide the child with a safe environment and a trusted adult where he or she can talk.
- Encourage the child to talk about what he or she has experienced, avoiding any "suggestions" or "leading questions".

- Avoid displaying "alarming emotions", which may prevent the child from relating factually correct information.
- Reassure the child that he or she did nothing wrong.
- Identify mental health facilities and professionals to help the child (psychologist, psychiatrist, or psychiatric social worker).
- Identify experienced pediatricians for a medical examination. (RATHUS, 2008).

Turn to Appendix I of this book for child abuse related resources recommended by the American Psychological Association.

Disorders related to *psychopathology* (abnormal behavior) are covered in a separate chapter in this book. However, because of much current concerns about autism, this disorder is being addressed here as well. The term *autism spectrum disorders* (ASDs), also known as *pervasive developmental disorders* includes autism, Asperger's syndrome, Rett's disorder, and childhood disintegrative disorder. Common symptoms of these disorders include repetitive stereotyped behavior, impaired social interaction, and poor communication skills. Sometimes these symptoms become noticeable by the end of the first year of life, but definitely by the age of three years (Butcher, Mineka, & Hooley, 2007). These disorders have become alarmingly common. According to the Centers for Disease Control (CDC) about one in every 152 children in the United States has an ASD (Rice, 2007). The present discussion will focus on autism. The three other related disorders are discussed in a separate section.

What exactly is *autism*? The most obvious feature of autism is a quality of "being alone", or "inward orientation". Frequent avoidance of eye contact, and persistent withdrawal from social interactions, and difficulty establishing emotional ties are the hallmarks of this serious disorder. Other characteristic symptoms include communication problems, intolerance of environmental changes and repetitive stereotypical behavior. These children shy away from parental attempt at affectionate contacts such as kissing or hugging. Speech development is delayed, and when it does appear around middle childhood, it is unusual and often difficult to understand. Children with autism are very "routine bound", and even minor deviations in daily activities may cause them visible distress often in the form of temper tantrums. They may even insist on eating the same food every day. In day care centers and schools they prefer keeping busy by themselves, rejecting attempts at peer involvement. Their emotional expression is restricted. They manifest deficits in imitative behavior and imaginative play. They often have reduced need for sleep (Butcher, Mineka, & Hooley, 2007). Some of their behavior is reminiscent of those seen in profoundly retarded children, such as self-mutilation in the form of repeated head banging, hand biting and hair pulling.

What do we know about the origins of autism spectrum disorders? Boys become victims of this disorder four to five times more frequently than girls. Some theorists claim that autism is a reaction to parental rejection. Empirical research *does not* support this theory. Mothers and fathers of autistic children are not deficient in parenting skills, and are able to express love and positive emotions. Most research results point to *biological* explanations for autism. It is believed that advanced maternal age and very low birth weight are associated with the risk of autism (Maimburg & Væth, 2006). High *concordance* (agreement) rates in *monozygotic* (identical) twin studies indicate genetic predispositions to this anomaly. Multiple genes are probably involved (Rutter, 2005). *Electroencephalographic* (brain wave) measures indicate abnormalities in the electrical activity and seizures in the brains of these children. Abnormal sensitivities to neurotransmitters (chemicals needed for normal brain functions) such as serotonin, dopamine, acetylcholine and norepinephrine have been detected as well (Bauman et.al, 2006; Cook, 1990). Unusually slow brain activities have been found in various parts of the brain. Some researchers implicate prenatal immune system involvement in this disorder (Zimmerman, Connors, & Prado-Villamizar, 2006). There has been some widespread belief that either vaccines, or the mercury preservative used in vaccines is the cause of autism. It is important to note, that there is *no* scientific evidence whatsoever to support this belief (Dales, Hammer, & Smith, 2001). The current professional view is that autism is a brain disease, *unrelated* in its etiology to vaccinations or parental influences.

What types of treatment are available to address autism? *Behavior modification* employing a variety of rewards and praises has been widely used to increase the child's ability to interact with others, and to reduce the frequency of self-mutilation. Parents are also involved in the process of therapy. Intensive *Individualized instruction* (over forty hours a week) has been used successfully to correct a variety of deficits related to autism. This method is quite rigorous and continuous, and often results in lasting improvements in communication skills and educational achievements (Lovaas, 2003). Pharmacological (medication) approaches have been successful in reducing aggressive and self-injurious behaviors. Drug treatment has also been used for the relief of anxiety, depression, and repetitive behaviors related to autism. These medications enhance serotonin activity in the brain (Kwok, 2003). Research centers around the world are working on improved understanding of the causes and treatment options for this devastating disorder.

It is important to realize that autism, like most mental and neurological illnesses, is manifested in different degrees of severity, and in different types and combinations of symptoms. Responses to treatment efforts are very individual as well. Although autistic behavior is ordinarily a lifelong condition, some autistic children can expect to graduate college, and trade schools, learn complicated skills, follow a career path, and live independently. The more severe cases require continuous treatment, specialized care or institutionalization. It is important for parents to recognize the early symptoms of autism, and to seek highly experienced professional help as quickly as possible.

When we talk about social and emotional development in infancy, the topic of *day care* is usually addressed. Day care is a "hot" topic nowadays, because the conventional way of raising children has been fading away. The desire of women to gain formal higher education and to aim for a career in life has altered child-rearing practices. Most mothers, including those with infants, have joined the workforce. In many cases economic circumstances have forced mothers to take part time or full time jobs. Consequently the difficult task of selecting appropriate day care facilities has become a reality in most American homes. Developmental experts have studied the various psychological effects that day care may have on children. The processes of attachment, social and cognitive development have been addressed. Some investigators reported that infants placed in full-time day care before twelve months of age may become insecurely attached to their parents (Belsky, 2001). According to highly reliable United States governmental studies however, such is not the case. The quality of day care facilities is a decisive factor in infants' social and emotional development. Infants with good quality day care experience rarely display insecure attachment to their mothers or fathers. Furthermore, they often demonstrate superior social behavior when compared to home-reared infants. Day care infants are more accustomed to social life. They feel more at ease with their peer group. They learn earlier how to communicate with peers, how to share toys, how to take turns in games, and how to react to others' feelings. Children in good quality centers are often affectionate, outgoing, display independent behavior, and self-confidence (Lamb & Ahnert, 2006). They feel comfortable in their interaction with both their peers and adults.

High quality day care has a positive effect on cognitive development, such as vocabulary, language and communication. There is also an association between day care exposure and better elementary school performance (Belsky, 2006). Children in day care centers often enjoy a better cognitive foundation for academic readiness. They are also better prepared emotionally to be away from their parents for extended time periods. Hence the transition to school life becomes less stressful. What constitutes a "high quality" day care center? A rich learning environment with ample availability of books, educational toys and instruments is important. A high ratio of caregivers to children is essential. The nature of interaction between children and caregivers is a significant determinant as well. It is preferred for caregivers to be educated, and to be fluent in grammatically correct

English. Day care staff should be motivated in their work, and should readily engage children in discussions and creative play activities. The physical environment also needs to have basic qualities, such as sufficient, clean and safe area for playing and active social interaction, appropriate lighting, coloration, furniture and pleasant decoration. Finding proper day care is a complicated process. Appendix II gives you some guidance related to this matter. (RATHUS, 247)

During the course of the first few months of development infants show only a limited number of emotions. There are two major theoretical positions on the development of emotions in infants. In 1932 Katherine Bridges theorized that babies are born with a single emotion, and other emotions become differentiated as the infant matures. In 2004 Carroll Izard posited that the major emotions are already present and even differentiated at the time of birth. These emotions however, are only manifested when they become needed in the maturational process. There is general agreement in the literature that emotional development is associated with both cognitive development and social exposure and experience. The expressions of fear, anger and joy have been seen in young infants.

Stranger anxiety (fear of strangers) has been extensively studied. The fear of strangers emerges between six and nine months of age. This is a normal developmental event, seen in many cultures, which has evolutionarily derived self-protective purposes. This type of fear protects animals from predatory advances, and protects children from potential harm by unfamiliar individuals. It is interesting to note that such anxiety is quite variable among children. Those children who have experience with adult interaction, such as seen in day care facilities, show less stranger anxiety. It has also been observed that strange children and women elicit less fear than strange men. Voice quality, facial features and body size may be influencing factors. When their mothers are present, children show less fear of strangers. When they are in familiar surroundings such as their homes, they also show less anxiety. When strangers touch them, their fear response dramatically increases (Boccia & Campos, 1989). When unfamiliar adults, such as a new friend of the family or a relative who rarely visits, attempt to befriend an infant it is important to be gentle and gradual. At first friendly and soothing talk from a distance is advisable. Offering toys, smiling, and engaging in playful gestures will reduce a child's anxiety. Passive and quiet behavior on the part of the unfamiliar adult may generate distress in infants probably because such "neutral" behaviors are difficult to interpret. Only after the establishment of a positive emotional contact, should infants be touched or picked up. In the third year of life stranger anxiety gradually declines.

Between six and eight months of age another interesting aspect of emotional development sets in. It is called *social referencing*. This process allows infants to use another person's reaction to a situation (usually an unfamiliar or ambiguous situation) to form their own assessment of it. For example, infants will be friendlier to a stranger when their mothers, or familiar caretakers appear relaxed and display a friendly attitude in the stranger's presence rather than a puzzled or worried facial expression (Stenberg, 2009). *Emotional regulation* is another important developmental event. This refers to the manner in which infants control their own emotional states. Research in this area indicates that children of secure mothers are able to manage their own emotions in a positive manner. Consistent two-way eye-to-eye communication with caregivers facilitates the development of appropriate emotional regulation. Securely attached infants are better able to regulate their emotions than those who are insecurely attached. According to some studies the quality of attachment in infancy has significant effects on emotional regulation later in life. For example, adolescents who enjoyed a secure attachment during their early years of development were better able to regulate their emotions and form cooperative friendly social relationships at ages sixteen and seventeen (Zimmermann et al., 2001).

Personality refers to a wide range of enduring, stable and important aspects of behavior. Personality traits are manifested in a predictable manner across many situations, and become characteristic of individuals. For example a "shy and introverted" person will most likely be shy in most unfamiliar social situations, and will be reluctant to initiate conversations. Some aspects of personality are unobservable. These may include our private ideas, thoughts, dreams or memories. The overt aspects of personality include physical actions, social interactions, communication styles, and many other observable behaviors.

Personality development begins with the emergence of the *self-concept*. This means self-awareness, or the impression that we have of ourselves. At birth babies have no realization that their bodies are entities separate from the surrounding environment. Gradually during infancy babies begin to realize that their hands and feet "belong" to them. They slowly develop a sense of self as they learn the details of their physical being and the space they occupy. They also begin to differentiate between their physical being and the selves of others. Self-awareness paves the road to social and emotional development. Positive social behaviors such as sharing and cooperation with peers are much dependent on the knowledge of the self. The experience of emotions such as shame, empathy, guilt, and embarrassment are also connected to self-knowledge (Foley, 2006). There are many theories of personality, as well as theories related to the development of personality. Appendix III describes several major personality theories.

Both genetic and environmental influences affect personality development. Some theories, such as the psychoanalytic view, first developed by Sigmund Freud around the year 1990, describe personality development in distinct stages. Freud stated that personality development consists of a series of *psychosexual stages*. A particular *erotogenic zone* (a body area associated with sexual pleasure) that serves as the primary source of pleasure characterizes each stage. The *Oral Stage (the first stage)* emerges during the first twelve to eighteen months of life. During this stage the infant's sexual desires center around the oral region, such as the mouth, the tongue and lips. While sucking at the breast or bottle provides nourishment and pleasure, frustrations may set in when food is not available immediately when the child is hungry. Furthermore, the child must eventually be weaned from the breast. Freud noted that the process of weaning is the first "lesson" the baby needs to learn about the sublimation (redirection) of instinctual urges and the satisfaction of the demands of society (Ewen, 2003).

Another leading psychodynamic theorist, Erik Erikson, posited that it is during the oral stage that interpersonal trust and mistrust develops. Parental attention and consistency is emphasized. A hungry infant will develop a trusting relationship with his caretaker if his needs are attended to in a timely and consistent manner. For example, food must be available in a consistent and predictable manner when a baby is hungry. When this is not the case, and the baby is ignored, and food is not supplied in a predictable fashion, the infant will develop a mistrustful relationship with his caretaker. Basic trust and mistrust, according to Erikson, has future consequences in forming social relationships in life. The child's increasing sense of becoming separate from and independent of the mother is called *separation-individuation*, a term coined by the famous psychoanalyst Margaret Mahler. This process begins at around five months and ends about three years of age (Mahler, Pine, & Bergman, 1975). The development of a healthy self-concept is very much the product of successful separation-individuation. This increasing sense of independence, autonomy, and control is demonstrated by repeated refusal to comply with parental directions and requests. This resistance, no matter how natural and normal, often becomes a source of frustration for parents. Nevertheless, children at all ages need to be given the opportunity to explore and to gradually find their way to an increased sense of independence. *Temperament* is a component of personality. Many personality theorists believe that temperament is genetically determined and remains stable throughout the developmental years and even extending to adulthood. It is a style of reaction, starting early in life, to environmental changes or to distinct stimuli. Researchers have identified the following characteristics of temperament:

- Activity level
- Smiling/laughter
- Regularity in child's biological functions, such as eating and sleeping
- Approach or withdrawal from new situations and people
- Adaptability to new situations
- Sensitivity to sensory stimulation

- Intensity of responsiveness
- Quality of mood—generally cheerful or unpleasant
- Distractibility
- Attention span and persistence
- Soothability
- Distress at limitations
  (Gartstein, Slobotskaya, & Kinsht, 2003; Thomas & Chess, 1989)

Studies in temperamental development indicate that children usually fall into one of three general categories shortly after birth. The "easy" child conforms easily to regular feeding and sleep schedules as set by parents. They show no resistance to new situations (new food, activity or people) and readily adapt to them. They are generally in a good mood. The "difficult" child does not conform well to established sleep and feeding schedules. They reluctantly accept new people and situations. They often initially resist new routines, and have little tolerance for frustration. They may burst out in violent crying and tantrums when faced with events which upset them. The "slow-to-warm-up" child shares some of the characteristics of the "difficult" child, but to a lesser degree (Thomas & Chess, 1989). Longitudinal studies (the same group of children are studied at various stages of development) have shown that "difficult" infants later on display antisocial behaviors, such as aggression in school. According to their teachers, their attention span is often shorter than average. Several studies have shown that children with temperamental problems are at greater risk for developing a variety of social adjustment difficulties and pathological behaviors later in life (Rothbart, Posner, & Hershey, 1995).

What can parents do to modify their children's biologically determined temperamental characteristics? To begin with, it is important for parents to understand and believe that children are at the "mercy" of their temperaments. They did not choose their personality traits, nor can they change it. Their "difficult" behavior is not intentional. Parents ought not to blame their children or themselves for these behavioral aberrations. Given this understanding, parents need to modify their expectations and curtail their own natural reactions to difficult children. These natural reactions include expressing frustration, being less available, less responsive, and ignoring their children's requests. Parents frequently have the attitude of "not wanting to be bothered", because they anticipate being nagged and annoyed by the "difficult" child. They may institute a punitive home environment, with rigid rules and schedules. They are often angry and short-tempered in their interaction with their children. Needless to say, this approach is counterproductive, and may result in more resistance and opposition on the part of the child. So, what to do? Parents need to learn to anticipate active resistance on the part of their children when they are faced with "new situations". New situations include, but are not limited to new rules and limits, new foods, new people, new games, new sounds, new activities, even if they are intended to be fun, such as birthday parties. Introduction to nursery or elementary school will also evoke violent protestations. Novel situations need to be introduced in a slow and gradual fashion, one at a time. Repeated exposure to novelty will eventually result in acceptance and accommodation on the part of the child. Children most often end up enjoying the new situation following a patient and incremental approach. Hence parents need to adjust their own behavior to their children's personality needs. This of course is not always an easy process, and parents may need professional guidance when faced with frustrating demands. Clinical child psychologists are well trained in the management of "difficult" infants and children. Appropriate parenting methods can modify to a certain degree children's temperamental difficulties, and may prevent adjustment problems later in life.

Parents and caretakers have a major role in teaching their children sex-appropriate behaviors. These behaviors become part of infants' personality structure, and continue to be shaped throughout their developmental years. Certainly, adults respond differently to girls and boys. Parents encourage boys to play with "masculine" toys, such as trucks and cars. Girls on the other hand are expected to play with dolls and dollhouses. Boys are dressed in "boy's colors", such as blue or brown. Girls are clad in pink and red. Boys are encouraged, especially by their fathers, to engage in more physical activities, whereas girls are expected to be gentle and cuddly. Research evidence indicates that by about two years of age both boys and girls seem to be able to appreciate the type of behaviors which are appropriate for their particular gender (Hill & Flom, 2007).

SECTION 1.5:
PHYSICAL DEVELOPMENT IN EARLY CHILDHOOD

The following topics are discussed in this section:
Growing patterns in early childhood
Physical development of the brain, and related psychological and motor functions
The capacity of the brain to heal itself
The relationship of handedness to physical and cognitive functions
Vaccinations, health and nutrition
How to minimize the risk for lead poisoning

Early childhood corresponds to ages two to six years. These are the preschool years. As compared to a child's infancy period, the growth rate proceeds slower during the preschool years. Throughout early childhood children tend to gain about two to three inches in height. They gain approximately four to six pounds per year. As they slowly lose their "baby fat", both boys and girls become noticeably slender (Rathus, 2008). The child's brain undergoes rapid development between two and six years of age. In normally developing children, by age six the brain will have reached about 90 percent of its adult weight. The process of myelination (the coating of neurons with a fatty insulating substance, permitting more rapid transmission of neural impulses) accounts partially to this rapid brain development. This process is particularly important with regard to the *cerebellum* (the part of the hindbrain involved in muscle coordination and balance). The development of fine motor skills is much dependent upon the myelination of the neural connections between the cerebellum and the cerebral cortex (the part of the brain involved with intellectual and voluntary motor functions) located in the forebrain (Nelson & Luciana, 2001). The ability to pay attention, to screen out distracting stimuli, and to process visual information, such as reading is also linked to the myelination process. These cognitive developments are necessary to meet the demands of schoolwork. Rapid growth in the frontal lobe and the left hemisphere of the brain allow for inhibition of responses, organizing and planning behavior, and continuous language development.

Sometimes we hear people to be characterized as "right-brained" or "left-brained". What exactly does this mean with regard to the neurological organization of the brain? Research in *neuropsychology* (the study of the relationship between the brain and behavior) suggests that in right-handed individuals the *left hemisphere* (left side) of the cerebrum is primarily involved with intellectual functions such expressive and receptive language skills, logic related to problem solving, and number concepts. The *right hemisphere* on the other hand, is usually better equipped for tasks related to visual-spatial functions such as solving puzzles, following maps, creative drawing, color discrimination, recognizing facial features, and facially expressed emotions, and body language. It is *not* true, however that some children are strictly right-brained and others are left-brained. The reason behind this is that brain function is not precisely divided between the two hemispheres. Some intellectual functions are shared between the two halves of the cerebrum. The right and left hemispheres can communicate with each other. This "sharing" function is further facilitated by the myelination of the *corpus callosum*, a thick bundle of nerve fibers which serve as a bridge to physically connect the two hemispheres (Kinsbourne, 2003). Children's improved ability to integrate emotional and logical functioning including perception, memory, attention, and problem solving is predicated on the continued myelination of the corpus callosum. The smooth coordination of physical movement is also associated with the corpus callosum.

Various brain imaging techniques and neuropsychological testing have taught us that the brain has many parts with specialized functions. Injuries to certain parts of the brain can result in the loss of abilities associated with these parts. Brain cells which constitute tissue do not regenerate, but certain mechanisms are available to compensate for injuries to particular neuroanatomical areas. The process of *"sprouting"* is partially responsible for this brain capacity. Sprouting involves the growth of new dendrites (projecting structures

38

of a nerve cell that receive impulses from neighboring nerve cells). This tendency of new parts of the brain to take over the functions of injured parts is called *plasticity*. This brain property is at its peak in very young children. After the second year of life plasticity gradually declines, but usually does not completely disappear even through adulthood (Kolb & Gibb, 2007). For example, if as a result of brain damage following a car accident a young child partially loses the ability to communicate, other brain areas may take over lost language functions, and the child will again be able to express himself and understand language. If an adult suffers this kind of brain damage, recovery will be very slow, and in most cases incomplete even with intense rehabilitative efforts.

Gross motor skills are those, which employ the large muscles. Examples are the use of arms for climbing, and legs for walking. Gross motor skills develop noticeably during the preschool years. Practice and motivation are important in learning various physical skills such as pedaling, kicking and throwing. Genetic predisposition related to muscular strength and coordination also plays an important role in the fine-tuning of gross motor skills. Children differ widely in their preferences and motivation for physical activity. Some prefer group activities, such as team sports and games, others like more solitary involvements, such as riding a tricycle. Some are more active than others. Active parents often have active children. The parental modeling of an active lifestyle with frequent outings and outdoor activities such as hiking, skiing, and ball playing, have a significant positive healthy effect on children.

Fine motor skills involve small muscles. The ability to move fingers and wrists in various directions are examples. Activities such as buttoning a shirt, zipping a jacket, and tying shoelaces require fine motor development. Many children enjoy drawing. The perfection of drawing involves both motor and cognitive skills. By the age of three, most children are able to draw a variety of basic shapes such as rectangles, crosses, circles and squares. Between the ages of four and five children's designs begin to be more sophisticated as they attempt to produce recognizable objects (Rathus, 2008). Drawing ability is also much dependent on practice and motivation. Parental encouragement can make a big difference. Both genetics and practice contribute to the development *handedness*, the tendency to prefer using the left or right hand in writing and other activities. If both parents are left-handed, the child's chances of being left–handed are about 50% (Annett, 1999). The bias in newborns' head position also contributes to hand preference. As a baby spends much time fixating and using on one hand, that particular hand will become more skillful over time (Hinojosa, Sheu, & Michael, 2003).

Much research has been conducted in the area of handedness. Approximately 10% of the general population is left-handed. There are both advantages and disadvantages to left-handedness. Above average mathematical skills, success in a number of athletic abilities (handball, boxing, basketball, baseball, fencing), and art fields (painters and musicians) have been associated with left-handedness (Coren, 1992). On the negative side, left-handedness has been associated with *dyslexia* (a reading disorder which may involve problems such as slow reading, letter reversals and reduced comprehension), stuttering, high blood pressure, epilepsy, depression and schizophrenia (Annett & Moran, 2006; Bryden, Broyn, & Fletcher, 2005). It is important to note that studies related to handedness are correlational. Cause and effect relationships between handedness and other factors should not be assumed.

Physical development is very much affected by nutritional factors. Well balanced diets (proteins, carbohydrates, fats, minerals, and vitamins) with appropriate caloric intake, support growth and energy requirements. As children advance in age their food requirements change. As the rate of physical growth declines in the preschool years, there is a decrease in appetite as well. The average child between the ages of four and six requires about 1400 calories per day (American Academy of Family Physicians, 2006). Childhood obesity needs to be prevented with the institution of healthful food preparation, supervised eating practices, and physical activities.

Children's appetite is often erratic. They may not be hungry at certain meals, and excessively hungry at others. There may be times when children will eat only very small amounts of food. This may be a source of concern for a mother. But the fact is that under ordinary conditions children will not starve themselves. They naturally regulate their food requirements. They may develop certain strange food preferences, or avoid certain foods altogether. It is not advisable to "force" children to eat certain types of foods or specified quantities of foods. Taste preferences often change in the developmental progression. Punishment for food refusal should also be avoided. Such tactics often result in anxiety and aversion related to eating. At times parents become frustrated when a child will refuse to eat a carefully prepared good-tasting healthy dish. Unfortunately this kind of behavior is normal and needs to be expected. It is wise to introduce new foods and flavors gradually, and in small quantities, until the child gets familiar with the textures, taste and odor of the novel dish. Over time, children's eating habits stabilize. In extreme cases consultation with a nutritionist is advised. Parents need to remember that as is the case with most learned behaviors, intentional or unintentional modeling of eating behaviors has lasting effects. For example if a father happens to be a "junk-food" eater, the likelihood is great that his child will also develop a preference for the kind of snacks he sees his father eat.

As we talk about physical development in early childhood, health and illness topics need to be briefly reviewed. Most children come down with at least some minor illnesses, and some with more serious maladies. It is advisable for parents to select pediatricians with whom both they and their children are comfortable. Visits to the doctor's office are usually anxiety-provoking events for most children. Hence a positive and friendly rapport between doctor, nurse and child will often allay feelings of tension. Parents need to feel free to ask pertinent questions related to their children's well being. Competent pediatricians and pediatric nurses will educate parents about proper health care, including topics such as nutrition, early symptom recognition and immunizations. Informative brochures are often available as well. Some minor illnesses include respiratory infections, such as colds, ear infections, and gastrointestinal irregularities, such as nausea, vomiting, and diarrhea. While these sicknesses cause discomfort and require medical attention, they do have some long-term beneficial effects, such as the creation of antibodies, which may protect children from developing these illnesses with further complications later in adulthood (Rathus, 2008).

Preventive measures need to be taken with regard to major childhood diseases. Appendix IV lists the diseases that childhood vaccines prevent. Precise vaccination schedules for children must be secured from pediatricians. Side effects such as slight fever, rash, and soreness at the site of the injection can be expected. Serious reactions to vaccinations are extremely rare, but if they do occur, the child must receive medical attention immediately. Continued medical and rehabilitative care is needed for children who suffer from chronic illnesses such as arthritis, diabetes, cerebral palsy, cystic fibrosis, cancer, asthma, and migraine headaches. Lead poisoning in childhood is a serious concern. High levels of lead in the body can cause irreversible neurological damage and behavioral disorders. These include lowered IQ, learning disabilities, distractibility, overactivity, antisocial behavior, headaches, auditory problems, and slow growth rate (Nevin, 2000). Appendix V lists suggestions for minimizing the risk of lead poisoning.

We may be surprised to learn that accidents are the most common cause of death in early childhood. Motor vehicle accidents are the leading cause, followed by drowning and fires. Boys, because of their generally more vigorous activities, are more at risk than girls. Preventive measures include the use of child safety seats in automobiles, installation of window guards in apartment buildings, use of safe toys fireproof clothing, and safe arrangements of furniture at home. Using common sense, some foresight and vigilant supervision are perhaps the most effective deterrents to accidental injuries.

Sleep is important for optimal physical and mental functioning. In their preschool years most children sleep between ten and eleven hours in a twenty-four hour period. This includes a daytime nap of one to two hours. Children frequently resist sleeping, especially in the evenings. This may be caused by stress related to separating from parents, or fear of darkness, or frightening dreams. Some researchers suggest that children should sleep together with their parents in the same bed, or at least in the same room to prevent sleep resistance. Others claim that co-sleeping may result in emotional problems such as excessive dependency, and foster habits which may be difficult to break, as the child gets older. Research results and professional opinions in this area are rather controversial. Suffocation may pose a danger if parents accidentally roll over their child as they sleep. For a variety of reasons some children develop sleep disorders. These are discussed in a separate chapter together with other pediatric psychological disorders.

The following topics are discussed in this section:
Determinants of intellectual development
The interaction of memory, motivation, emotion, and cognitive organization
The development of vocabulary, grammar, and pragmatics in early childhood

Between the ages of two to seven years important intellectual changes occur. Jean Piaget (the famous child psychologist) stated that in the course of these years, the preoperational stage, children's thought processes are characterized by the use of symbols to represent objects and events. The use of language is an important example of symbolic activity. Expression in the form of drawings is another example. *Symbolic play*, also known as "pretend play" is a hallmark of this cognitive developmental period. When engaged in symbolic play, children make believe that objects and toys represent something other than what they really are (Piaget, 1962; Smith, Cowie, & Blades, 2003). Examples of pretend play include activities such as a little boy pretending that he is a doctor as he is "examining" the heartbeat of a friend with a toy stethoscope. Similarly a little girl may take her doll for a walk in a toy baby carriage. The nature of pretend play is predictive of future behavioral qualities. Friendly, kind, constructive, and elaborate pretend play activities often result in better peer relationships, school performance, and creativity. Aggressive and violent symbolic play produces less empathy and more tendencies for antisocial acts in later development (Dunn & Hughes, 2001).

Egocentrism is another salient aspect of the preoperational stage. This characteristic refers to children's inability to understand that people may have opinions, views, and perspectives other than their own. In other words, they can only see events from their own particular point of view. This is a consequence of inflexible one-dimensional thinking, which is typical at this stage of development. *Precausal* thinking involves an egocentric type of reasoning. For example, the question, "Why does it rain?" would receive an answer, such as, "Because the rain wants to water the plants." The question, "Why does it get light outside in the morning?" would receive the answer, "Because I have to get up in the morning". *Animism* and *artificialism* are also often seen in preoperational children. Animism is the attribution of life and intentionality to inanimate objects. For example, as a three-year-old child gets out of the car in a large garage, he may comment, "The cars are all sleeping." Artificialism is the belief that aspects of the environment were created by people. For example, "The sky is blue because someone painted them that color" (Smith, Cowie, & Blades, 2003; Shaffer, 2002). There is also the tendency at this age for children to believe that dreams are real, and that others can see their dreams because dreams come form the outside. It is for this reason that young children are often afraid to go to sleep at night. In some cases insomnia may develop.

Centration and *irreversibility* are two other aspects of preoperational thinking. Centration is the inability to focus on more than one dimension of a problem at a time. Irreversibility speaks to the lack of recognition that actions can be reversed. The physical law of "conservation" tells us that properties of substances such as volume, mass or quantity remain the same even if we change their arrangement. For example the amount of play dough will remain the same regardless of its changing shape. Similarly, the amount of liquid remains the same regardless of the change in the shape of the container in which it is stored (Shaffer, 2002). Young children have difficulties appreciating this concept. All of the aforementioned cognitive "irregularities" are normal, and will be corrected as a function of the maturation of the brain, and education of the child.

There are a number of factors, which positively affect cognitive development in children. These include the parents' educational level, active verbal and emotional communication of parents with their children, emotionally stable and stimulating home environment including access to creative play materials, books and educational television programs. Physical and mental illness of parents, financial stress in the family, excessive punitive methods, and divorce have negative effects. Preschool education for economically disadvantaged children such as Head Start programs have beneficial effects on later school performance, social adjustment, and career success.

What is the *theory of mind*? This is a concept that we as adults rarely, if ever, think about. It has to do with our basic understanding of how the mind works (Feldman, 2012). It is a familiarity with our thought processes, and the interaction between our emotional states, cognitive processes, and behavior. Knowing how the mind works allows us to better appreciate our perceptions, and the behavior of those around us. It also helps us predict the reactions of others to us, and to better distinguish appearance from reality in our daily environmental encounters. Preschool children gradually acquire the capacity to understand how we acquire knowledge and the interaction among our sensory modalities. For example, an orange has an identifiable shape that can be seen, a texture that can be felt, an odor that can be smelled, and a taste that can be tasted. Hence to correctly perceive an orange we need to use our eyes, hands and fingers, nose, and mouth. They also learn the meaning of deception and the ability to detect misleading information.

Preschool children have rather well developed memory skills. Both *recognition* and *recall* tasks have been used in memory research. Recognition tasks involve remembering previously experienced information upon seeing or hearing it again. Recall tasks offer no cues, and the individual needs to respond to questions from memory. Most children find recall more difficult than recognition. Factors, which influence memory, include what needs to be remembered, interest level of the child (motivation), retrieval cues, and the way memory is measured (Rathus, 2008). Research results suggest that at this age children's memories for activities are better than their memories for objects (Jones, Swift, & Johnson, 1988). For example, when a little girl is engaged in pretend play of "house and family", she will remember more readily the activities involved, such as "washing the baby" or "putting the baby to sleep" than the actual objects involved in the activities, such as the soap, washing cloth, or color of the doll's bed.

Researchers also tell us that preschool children show a preference for logical order when remembering events (Fivush, Kuebli, & Clubb, 1992). For instance a little girl will remember the order of events which took place as she was pretend playing "getting her 'daughter' ready for school in the morning". On the other hand, she will have difficulties remembering the *random* activities involved when playing ball in a park. Events, which are unusual and are associated with positive or negative emotional reactions, are easier to recall. For instance a child will easily remember details related to his birthday party if his favorite friends surrounded him, and if his gifts included toys he wanted to have for a long time. Similarly he will easily remember the movie he saw several weeks ago in California, when as he was watching the film, an earthquake was happening, and he had to leave the movie house.

All parents know how difficult it can be to get a child's attention when they are involved in something that interests them. In fact, *attention* is a significant aspect of memory. Furthermore, *motivation* often is the driving force behind attention. Motivation may be *intrinsic*, such as interest in playing with a new toy, or *extrinsic* such as helping mother do the dishes for the privilege of watching a favorite television show later on. Research indicates that interest level, motivation, and attention are major determinants of memory functions in preschool children (Ghetti & Alexander, 2004). Children at this age also have increasingly well developed *autobiographical memory* (memory for special events in their lives, such as a birthday party) (Wang, 2008). Retrieval cues, or hints also help children in their recall. It is useful for parents to provide such cues. Because language and communication ability are closely tied to memory, children at times may find it easier to reenact an event using dolls and other toy items than to give a verbal account of things remembered. Children can be taught simple memory strategies, such as rehearsal, which simply involves either mental or vocal repetition. Categorization is another method. For example, when trying to remember the types of wearing apparel we have in our closets, it may be useful to think of them in terms of summer and winter clothes, or formal (work) and informal (leisure) clothes.

During the preschool years children's language skills undergo very noticeable changes. Children become talkative, and readily engage themselves in conversations with their peers and caregivers. Advances in vocabulary, grammar, and pragmatics (the practical aspects of communication) facilitate correct language usage and expressive skills. As children begin to feel that others understand them, their motivation increases to further use and refine their language. Children in the preschool years rapidly increase their vocabulary; they learn approximately nine new words per day. Grammatically correct sentences using conjunctions (or, and , but), pronouns (he, her, they), articles (the, a, an), prepositions (over, under, behind, around), and possessive adjectives (our, their), are increasingly used. Passive sentences, such as "The baby was scratched by the cat" are rarely used correctly in early childhood (Feldman, 2012; Strohner & Nelson, 1974; Tamis-LaMonda et al., 2006). As children develop their linguistic skills parents are encouraged to pay close attention and correct their children's grammatical errors. Recognition and reward of proper language usage will further motivate children to communicate appropriately. Preschool children also begin to show the ability to alter their style of speech to fit specific social situations. For instance, they use different syntax (sentence structure) and words when they are faced with high-status individuals, such as teachers, elderly people, or their physicians, whom they wish to respect respect.

SECTION 1.7:
SOCIAL AND EMOTIONAL DEVELOPMENT
IN EARLY CHILDHOOD

The following topics are discussed in this section:
The influence of parents, siblings and peers on social and emotional development
How parents should use rewards and punishments effectively in an attempt to modify their children's behavior
The effects of birth order on behavior
The development of empathy and prosocial behavior
What parents can do to minimize children's aggressive behavior
The development of self-concept and self-esteem
The evolution of gender roles

Parents, siblings, and peers have important influences on children's social and emotional development. The quality of family life is an important determinant because preschool children spend much of their wakeful hours at home. There is a large body of research literature on patterns of child rearing. Two spectrums of parental characteristics have been studied: *warmth-coldness* and *restrictiveness-permissiveness* (Baumrind, 1989). *Warm* parents are emotionally expressive. They tend to hug and kiss their children. They often smile and act in a caring and supportive fashion. They convey a feeling of happiness and satisfaction with their children. They rarely use physical discipline. *Cold* parents, on the other hand are not very expressive emotionally. They do not communicate enjoyment in being with their sons and daughters. They make children feel that they are a burden. They often complain about their children's behavior, and describe them as naughty. They rarely praise them or pay attention to their positive qualities. Children who grow up in an accepting and warm environment are more likely to internalize socially desirable manners of behavior, and a sense of moral correctness. They will also likely enjoy positive social and emotional adjustment. Parents' attitude toward their children often reflects their past experiences in their own parental homes as they grew up.

Restrictive parents are vigilant and enforce rules, which are designed to prevent accidents and injuries in the home, in the playground, in the car, or on trips to places such as museums or the zoo. Child psychologists agree that sensible, consistent control of inappropriate or potentially dangerous behaviors has positive effects on children. Such control should be delivered in a supportive and caring manner, with explanations, avoiding excessive restrictions and harsh punitive measures; when possible, desirable behaviors should be recognized and rewarded. *Permissive* parents follow the philosophy of "laissez-faire", allowing children to act out their natural tendencies with minimal interference. They allow children to be noisy, messy and somewhat disrespectful toward others, and toward their environment and possessions. For instance throwing and breaking toys will have no consequences. Permissive parents are not necessarily negligent. They believe that children need freedom of expression in their young formative years. Some research evidence support permissive parents' beliefs. Correlations were reported between permissive parenting styles, positive self-esteem, and psychological adjustment (Martinez et al., 2003).

Studies have focused on three types of methods used by parents to enforce rules and restrictions. *Inductive techniques* involve reasoning and explanations related to rules and regulations. Parents attempt to be reasonable with the hope that their children will understand the logic behind restrictive measures. Children who are open to such explanations will not feel that their freedom is curtailed unnecessarily, and may comply more willingly with the restrictions imposed upon them. *Power-assertive methods* often have a variety of negative consequences. Power assertion includes harsh physical punishment with little or no explanations, and denial of privileges, such as playing with friends, using the telephone or watching television. Children who are exposed to these methods frequently become rebellious and non-compliant. Their school performance is negatively affected and they tend to be aggressive and engage in antisocial behaviors.

Withdrawal of love is the third method. Parents may say to their sons and daughters: "I will not love you if you do not listen to what I am telling you.", or they may simply ignore their children and assume a non-responsive attitude. Children will often become anxious when faced with "silent treatment" and loss of affection. They need their parents' attention. Withdrawal of love can be perceived by children as more punitive than physical punishment; hence it results in compliant behavior, often accompanied by anxiety (Grusec, 2002). Positive approaches are often fruitful. Rather than saying: "You must stop listening to all that loud music", proposing a different activity may yield less resistance: "Let us invite your friend, Paul to play some board games".

Four *parenting styles* have been identified by research psychologists. These are, *authoritative, authoritarian, permissive-indulgent,* and *rejecting-neglecting.* Each of these styles has been associated with a variety of developmental consequences. The *authoritative* parenting style is the preferred one with regard to behavioral outcomes. Parents who adopt this style respect their children, and create a warm family environment with minimal tension. While they demand mature behavior with well-defined goals, they are supportive, and readily recognize their children's efforts. They avoid harsh punishment, and use reason in their interaction with their children. Sons and daughters of authoritative parents develop high self-esteem, self-reliance and independence. They are achievement oriented, socially competent, active, and willing to explore and learn. *Authoritarian* parents have a "military" approach to childrearing. They insist on obedience, and do not tolerate any challenges to the "rules of the house". The prevailing motto is "You do what I tell you, because I said so." They exercise forceful control, rather than supportive control. They rarely reason with their children, and show no respect for their children's viewpoints and achievements. They are cold and curt, and short on communicating positive emotions. The children of these parents are hostile and defiant. They rarely initiate activities, but rather follow their peers in social situations. They are less independent, show less social competence, lower self-esteem, and less academic success than children of authoritative parents. They are often anxious, irritable, and not very friendly.

Permissive-indulgent parents set only few "rules and regulations", and do not demand much obedience. While they are vigilant about safety issues, and may "childproof" their homes, the general attitude is "live and let live". Little attention is paid to respect, order, and goal setting. There often is a chaotic, disorganized home environment. These parents are warm, supportive, rarely punitive, and often encourage their children to be active and creative. The children of these parents are scholastically "average", and prone to misconduct. They are usually self-confident and socially competent (Cole, Cole & Lightfoot, 2005). *Rejecting-neglecting* parents are poorly responsive and non-supportive. There is a general sense of carelessness in their interaction with their children. They have few demands and display infrequent control, as if saying, "I don't want to be bothered". They are often unaware of potential hazards and may put their children at risk for accidents and injuries. They pay little attention to school related matters. Their children are often low academic achievers, and socially unprepared. They frequently show disciplinary problems and deviant behaviors such as substance abuse. Generally speaking, strict authoritarian methods as well as excessive permissiveness need to be avoided. Frustrated parents, who feel that their children understand the "dos" and the "don'ts", and who are capable of behaving properly, and who "purposefully" disregard rules, often resort to harsh punitive methods. Parents who are under a lot of stress may also turn to power assertive methods of control. Appendix VI lists some suggestions for parental guidance of young children.

It is important for parents to realize that siblings have significant influence on each other's behavior, as well as on social, cognitive and emotional development (McHale, Kim, & Whiteman, 2006). Hence they need to be taught positive cooperative behavior directly, and through modeling. Parents are advised to treat their children as individuals. While spending quality time as a "family" is important, each child deserves individual attention. Parents need to be familiar with their children's strengths, weaknesses, and preferences. They should not be expected to compete with each other on any level, but to respect, help, and appreciate each other.

Firstborn and only children enjoy a special status in the average family. They receive maximal attention, time and care. In the mind of a child the arrival of a new sibling may upset this special status, and realistically so. To minimize this perceived threat and associated anxieties parents need to carefully prepare their son or daughter for the arrival of the new baby. Expected changes in the mother's and father's responsibilities need to be discussed. The child needs to be reassured of continued support, love and care. Involving the child in the care of the baby is often helpful, and helps sow the seeds for an ongoing cooperative rather than competitive relationship.

Birth order has been extensively studied. Firstborn children are generally more achievement oriented than later-born children. They are more cooperative, helpful, and scholastically better students. They are also less aggressive and less self-reliant. Later-born children at times develop aggressive tendencies. Perhaps they feel the need to "fight" for attention and recognition. Their enhanced adaptive skills result in social success among their peers.

Play activities have a significant role in social and cognitive development. Children learn to share toys, take turn in games, experience how it feels to compete, win, and lose. They learn how to solve problems, and think symbolically. Jean Piaget proposed that play expresses milestones in cognitive development. He identified the following kinds of play: (Piaget, 1962).

- *Functional play.* This begins in the sensorimotor stage, and involves repetitive motor activities such as rolling a ball, or hitting a rattle.
- *Symbolic play.* Begins toward the end of the sensorimotor stage, and increases during early childhood. Children assume roles, create settings, characters and scripts (descriptions of behaviors in specific situations)
- *Constructive play.* During early childhood children use blocks to build, draw, paint, or make something out of paper or cardboard.

- *Formal games.* Children learn to follow rules using board games, or playing hopscotch. They learn how to interact in team competitions. They strategize and plan ahead. This is the most advanced and complex form of play.

There are obvious sex differences in play activities. Generally speaking boys tend to enjoy rough and vigorous physical outdoor activities during preschool and early elementary school years. Arts and crafts, as well as domestic play are the preferred activities for girls. Boys prefer the company of boys, and girls seek out other girls.

Altruistic (prosocial) behavior is defined as the kind of behavior which is intended to benefit another person without expectation of reward. By the preschool and early school years children often engage in this kind of helping behavior. *Empathy* is the ability to understand and share another person's feelings. It is the feeling of sorrow for another's plight. This includes interpersonal sensitivity and cooperation. As early as the second year of life children (girls more often than boys) show evidence of empathetic tendencies. Children who are skilled at regulating their emotions, and are sociable, are more likely to display prosocial behaviors such as sharing, helping and comforting others when the need arises (Bengtson, 2005). Prosocial behavior is learned. Rewarding prosocial behavior by peer acceptance and parental training and approval results in the continuance of such behaviors. Observing parents' helping behaviors and secure parental attachment enhance altruistic qualities in children (Clark & Ladd, 2000). Authoritative parenting styles foster helping behaviors.

Aggressive behavior has many negative social consequences. Aggression may be physical, verbal, or relational. Kicking, hitting or destroying another's property are examples of physical aggression. Verbal aggression involves teasing, threatening, or insulting others. Gossiping, and social exclusion are means of relational aggression. Children who intentionally hurt others are not readily accepted into the social network of their peers. Finding themselves socially excluded, their aggressive tendencies often increase. Later in life as they befriend other children with antisocial tendencies, they frequently engage themselves in criminal behaviors. The development of aggression has biological, cognitive and learning determinants. Genetics play a role as well. Elevated testosterone (male sex hormone) level and reduced levels of serotonin have been associated with aggressive behavior. Erroneous interpretation of peer behavior (incorrectly assuming peer hostility), lack of empathy, and the inability to see things from other people's point of view often trigger aggressive acts. Children who are exposed to hostile home environments and physical punishment frequently learn to resort to aggressive means in order to get their way. Violent movies and television programs also have a negative effect on children's behavior (Villani, 2001). As children join others who act aggressively, they mutually reinforce each other as they act out their negative social behaviors. Parents can take a variety of measures to minimize the development of aggressive behaviors in their sons and daughters:

1. Avoid violent physical and verbal fights at home.
2. Avoid the use of abusive language.
3. Avoid excessive physical punishment.
4. Reasons for punishment need careful explanation.
5. Model and teach prosocial behaviors to children.
6. Consistently reward socially correct behaviors such as sharing, being respectful, and being sensitive to other's feelings.
7. Detect and address children's perceived and actual frustrations.
8. Sensitize children to the consequences of aggressive behavior, including the negative effects of their behavior on others.
9. Teach children to understand other persons' perspectives.

The *self concept* (sense of self) develops during early childhood. Children begin to widen their understanding of who they are, how they feel about themselves, what they are capable of doing, and how they are different from others. They are aware of sex differences, and changes in their feelings as they encounter different situations, such as unfamiliar environments or strangers. They also appreciate behavioral states, such as "being scared" and "behaving bad". *Self esteem* is an important aspect of personality development. It is the extent to which an individual accepts and values the self. Positive feedback from others, and a sense of achievement have a favorable effect on self esteem. Mothers and fathers who practice authoritative style of parenting often have children with positive self-esteem. These children are securely attached and have caring and attentive parents (Booth-LaForce, et al., 2006). Parents can promote positive self-esteem development in their children by recognizing and rewarding their efforts and achievements.

Gender roles or *gender typing* refer to roles, activities, traits, or behaviors that are considered *stereotypical* (conventional) of males and females in a particular culture. Stereotypical activities in children develop early (around three years of age). Boys are often more aggressive and engage in physical play routines. Girls are more empathetic, and display better developed verbal abilities than boys. Visual-spatial abilities are better developed in boys. The behavioral expression of male-female sex differences has neurobiological, genetic, hormonal and social cognitive (children's observation of other's sex-linked behaviors) roots. Parental expectations, and the differential approval and rewarding of their children's behaviors play a significant part in the development of sex-linked activities in children. *Psychological androgyny* is the possession of a mixture of both stereotypical feminine and masculine traits. Results of a number of studies indicate that androgynous children are well adjusted because they possess both kinds of socially valued traits, which maximize their ability to successfully cope with a broader range of challenges which they face in their life. (Berk, 2013; Lefkowitz & Zeldow, 2006).

SECTION 1.8:
PHYSICAL DEVELOPMENT IN MIDDLE CHILDHOOD

The following topics are discussed in this section:
Physical development and nutrition
The psychological effects of obesity and poor physical fitness

In the course of middle childhood (seven to twelve years of age) children continue to gain about two inches in height per year. Over a five year period body weight doubles. Children are active both physically and mentally during this period. Academic demands increase, as well as social, and sports activities. Proper nutrition is important to support energy requirements. Approximately 2000 calories per day is needed. A well-balanced healthy diet is crucial. Parents are encouraged to model healthy eating behaviors. Children can easily acquire poor nutritional practices when watching their parents eat harmful food items, such as excessive sweets, salty snacks, or meals high in fats and carbohydrates. "Forbidden" food items should never be used as "rewards" for desired behaviors or achievements. Obesity in childhood has negative medical and psychological effects. Traditionally obesity has been determined by weight. Many researchers advocate a more accurate measure known as *body mass index* (BMI). This is the ratio of weight to height. The formula for the calculation of the BMI is as follows: *BMI = height in inches/weight in pounds² X 703.* Those boys and girls whose BMI falls between the 85th amd 95th percentile are considered at risk for obesity. Using this criterion, in our country approximately 15% of children ages 6 to 11 are overweight (American Academy of Pediatrics, 2003). Obesity in childhood may result in concurrent health complications and future abnormal conditions such as high blood pressure, heart disease, diabetes, and hardening of the arteries (Daniels, 2006). Furthermore, overweight children are frequently subjected to ridicule by their peers. Their inferior performance in sports and physical play activities results in social rejection and stigmatization. As they get older, they become less desirable to the opposite sex. Consequently their body image is poor, and their self-esteem is negatively affected. Heredity plays a very significant role in obesity. Children whose parents are overweight require special attention. Consulting a clinical nutritionist for preventive measures is highly recommended. The importance of establishing proper dietary habits in childhood cannot be overemphasized.

Poor eating practices are very difficult to break later in life, even with professional intervention. Sedentary life styles definitely contribute to weight gain. Spending long hours in front of a television set, or with a computer needs to be discouraged in a consistent fashion. Excessive food intake as a means of seeking psychological comfort is also associated with children's emotional state. Stress, anxiety and depression may contribute to eating. Frequent fights and arguments at home, unreasonable parental expectations, and coercive punitive tactics can cause stressful conditions for children, resulting in maladaptive eating habits. Physical, recreational and sport activities need to be regularly incorporated in children's weekly routines. Physical fitness often results in improved social adjustment and academic performance. Appendix VII lists suggestions for weight management.

Throughout middle childhood children's nervous system and musculature continue to develop. Both fine motor skills and gross motor skills, as well as reaction time improve accordingly. Sports, exercises, and physical play activities should be encouraged. Increased physical prowess leads to more self-sufficiency, exploration, independence, and interest in novel hobbies, such as sewing and knitting for girls, and woodwork projects for boys. Not all children develop at the same rate. Some sex differences are to be expected. In general boys' muscle mass exceeds that of girls. Periodic visits to the pediatrician are recommended to keep track of normal rates of physical development. Abnormal developmental lags and disabilities (e.g. speech, hearing, vision, learning) must be addressed professionally on a timely basis.

The brain also continues to develop significantly at this age. Myelination, and improved neural connections, especially in the frontal lobes facilitate more advanced cognitive processes, such as attention, planning and problem solving.

SECTION 1.9:
COGNITIVE DEVELOPMENT IN MIDDLE CHILDHOOD

The following topics are discussed in this section:
Cognitive flexibility and logic
Information processing
The mechanisms of memory
The definition of intelligence and intelligence quotient (IQ)
The meaning of emotional intelligence
Tests used to measure intelligence
Creativity
Moral development

Children's thought processes and language development undergo significant changes during this period. Middle childhood marks the stage of *concrete operations,* according Jean Piaget. Between the ages of seven and twelve children begin to show increased capacity for logic and cognitive flexibility. Their thinking, however mostly involve "concrete" (tangible) aspects of the environment, rather than concepts which are "abstract" in nature. They become familiar with concepts such as *reversibility* and the physical laws of *conservation.* Hence they can appreciate the arithmetical operations of addition and subtraction. They begin to understand that the amount or mass of a substance, such as play dough, will remain the same regardless of the shape it takes. They are also able to group objects according to certain physical properties, such as color, shape, height, or weight. This is called *seriation.* Relational logic also involves the concept of *transitivity,* which is the capacity to appreciate relations among elements in a serial order. For example if Jack is older than Jim, and Jim is older Bruce, than it follows that Jack has to be older than Bruce. *Another* cognitive skill is *class inclusion.* This involves categorization according to "classes" and "subclasses" (e.g. the subclasses of "dogs" and "cats" belong to the class of "animals", which in turn belong to the higher class of "living things", which also include "plants") (Shaffer, 2002).

The *information processing* approach to cognitive development examines processes such as attention, memory, and problem solving. One of the fundamental requirements for effective cognitive functioning is the ability to pay attention. The ability to focus, and to screen out irrelevant information is moderately well developed by middle childhood. This capacity is predicated on both biological (neurological) readiness and appropriate discipline. Over the years much research has been conducted in the area of memory. Scientists have differentiated among many types of memory. For our purposes a general overview of this subject matter will suffice. Most researchers propose that there are three major memory structures: sensory memory, working (short-term) memory, and long-term memory. *Sensory memory* maintains information for only a fraction of a second, before it decays. For example, as we walk on the street we notice many changing events around us, but most of what we see we promptly "forget". In order to prevent forgetting, we must pay attention to the stimuli which we encounter. Focusing facilitates remembering. When a child pays attention, information will be transferred from sensory memory to *working memory*. Visual information in working memory may be retained for about thirty seconds. Auditory information can be maintained longer, especially if the information is repeated (rehearsed). Preadolescent children can store between three to five chunks of information (such as telephone numbers) in working memory.

Long-term memory has unlimited storage capacity. The retrieval of information from long-term memory often requires certain "cues" before it can be accessed. Cues trigger the associations (related available information) which were employed when certain memories were originally stored. Long-term memory has a "preference" for meaningful information. Information which is poorly understood, or which has no personal significance will generally not be stored permanently. Emotionally meaningful material, such as severe punishments or personally relevant information (e.g. address, telephone number, date of birth) will readily be remembered. It therefore behooves both teachers and parents to encourage children to thoroughly comprehend newly learned topics and concepts which need to be memorized. In middle childhood children's ability to understand and differentiate among concepts significantly increases. Formal education, of course, facilitates this process. The placement of newly acquired information into long-term storage adheres to a categorization process. Conceptual categorization is essential for easy access when retrieval is attempted. For example, the appreciation of the concept of "dairy products" will facilitate the establishment of the "dairy" category. Consequently, all newly learned "milk products" will automatically be stored in this category. It naturally follows that when a child is asked to name from memory as many dairy products as he can, he will have an easy time doing this as he "opens up" this readily available category of information in his long-term memory. Here again we need to emphasize the importance of the understanding of newly learned information. Poorly understood information may either end up in the wrong category, and cause confusion upon recall, or may be lost from memory.

Metacognition is an interesting concept, we often do not think of. It has to do with our understanding and awareness of our own thinking processes. As children's understanding of their mind develops they can better control their cognitive abilities. Problem solving involves metacognition when we use differential techniques and strategies to arrive at solutions. Being aware of the mechanism of our memory system (*metamemory*), facilitates retention and retrieval of information. Rehearsals, associations, clustering, and categorization of newly learned material are examples of techniques used in memorization. Making children aware of such techniques will help them academically.

What is intelligence? And how do we measure it? These are probably the two most intriguing questions in the field of cognitive psychology. There are a variety of theories of intelligence. For our purposes a brief review of the better-known theories will suffice. *Intelligence*, in general implies the ability of an organism to *adapt* to environmental demands. Coping with environmental changes necessitates the understanding of what our world is all about, and how it operates. In order to exist successfully, we need to be familiar with both the physical and social aspects of our environment. Adaptability includes flexibility and sometimes also creativity. For example, to survive under climatic changes, our dressing behavior needs to be flexible. Successful adaptation to cultural changes requires flexibility in social behavior. Resorting to novel problem solving strategies requires cognitive flexibility and creativity. As is the case with many psychological processes, intelligence has both biological and learning components.

Repeatedly, research results suggest that genetics also plays a significant role in intellectual capacities. In 1904 Charles Spearman, a British psychologist viewed intelligence as the ability to reason and to solve problems. He believed that most intellectual functions are based on these two capacities. In 1938 the American psychologist, Louis Thurstone suggested that specific factors compose the concept of intelligence. He talked about abilities such as perceptual speed, visual-spatial, numerical, reasoning, vocabulary, and memory (Thurstone & Thurstone, 1941). Contemporary views of intelligence incorporate many of these factors. The theoretician, Robert Sternberg offered a more basic description. He divided intellectual abilities into three components: analytical, creative, and practical. Academic ability is related to analytical intelligence; the ability to solve novel problems, and to learn from experience depends on creative intelligence; adaptation to environmental demands requires practical intelligence (Sternberg, 1997). While the concept of "creative intelligence" has been debated in the literature, Sternberg's two other definitions have been mostly accepted by present-day psychologists.

In opposition to Sternberg, some psychologists believe that intelligence is a complicated multidimensional concept. Howard Gardner, for example envisioned intelligence as having nine elements: linguistic (verbal ability), spatial (visual-spatial skills), interpersonal (ability to relate to others and empathy), logical-mathematical (numerical reasoning), bodily-kinesthetic (athletics and dancing), intrapersonal (self-knowledge and insight), naturalist (understanding of natural events and the behavior of organisms living in nature), musical

(musical appreciation and talents), and existential (appreciation of philosophical issues in life) (Gardner, 1983). This presentation resembles a *neuropsychological* approach. Neuropsychology is the study of brain-behavior relationships. In fact Gardner believed that each aspect of intelligence, as described above, relates to specific brain areas. There is no strong scientific support for this assumption.

A relatively recent and widely accepted concept is *emotional intelligence*. Psychologists Peter Salovey and John Mayer developed this theory approximately fifteen year ago (Salovey & Pizarro, 2003). The concept involves insight and awareness of one's inner feelings, and sensitivity to the feelings of others. Emotional intelligence certainly complements the general definition of intelligence, because it has to do with necessary ingredients needed for effective interpersonal relationships. Paying attention to the effect our mood, tonality and body language has on others is important when trying to understand the reactions of others to our behavior. Self control, empathy, sensitivity to facially expressed messages, and the ability to see things from somebody else's viewpoint and emotional state are essential to successful social interactions in life. In summary, both academic skills and emotional awareness are essential for adaptive behavior.

Now that we have explored some of the major theories of intelligence, we are ready to introduce a related topic: the measurement of intelligence. Many American and other children around the world are subjected to intelligence testing. Such tests are often administered by clinical or school psychologists in the context of children's academic life. More precisely, intelligence tests are believed to be predictive of scholastic performance. Hence they are used to determine placement in a variety of academic settings. Slow learners and gifted children require special curricula to meet their intellectual needs. These tests are also used when there is a suspicion of learning disabilities or mental retardation. In conjunction with other *neuropsychological tests* (tests of cognitive abilities), intelligence tests are also administered to detect the possibility of brain damage in cases such as traumatic injuries, or dementia. The *Stanford-Binet Intelligence Scale* has a long history. It was originated in France about one hundred years ago. It was constructed in response to a need to identify children who could not benefit from regular classroom education in the French public school system. Since its original version, which was introduced in 1905, this test was modified several times. In 1916 this instrument was first used in the United States. Using this test, it became possible to compute a child's *intelligence quotient,* or *IQ.* By definition, the formula for the IQ is as follows: $IQ = \dfrac{\text{Mental Age (MA)}}{\text{Chronological Age (CA)}} \times 100.$

Mental age denotes the intellectual level at which a specific child is functioning. For example, a child whose mental age is eight, is said to be functioning at the level of an average eight-year-old child. According to the above formula, a child whose mental age is eight and chronological age is eight, will have an IQ of 100. Similarly, a child whose mental age is higher than his chronological age will have an IQ which is above a hundred; and a child whose mental age is below his chronological age, will have an IQ which is below 100. In 1939 *David Wechsler,* a psychologist in New York City, working at Bellevue Hospital, constructed an instrument for the measurement of intelligence in adults. This instrument is comprised of several sub-tests; some are intended to measure "verbal" tasks, others measure "performance" tasks. An IQ score can be computed for either sub-test, as well as for the entire test. Later on Wechsler also developed similar instruments for the measurement of school-age and younger children's intelligence (Wechsler, 1975). Appendix VIII describes in more detail the Stanford-Binet and Wechsler scales (Known as the WAIS or WISC).

Intelligence tests have been criticized on the grounds that they are *biased.* In other words, it is felt that one requires to have a certain type of cultural experience in order to score well on these tests. In an attempt to avoid this problem, psychologists have tried to construct culture-fair intelligence tests. These tests, however are poor predictors of academic success, hence their usefulness is limited.

Research results in this area tell us that level of intelligence is determined by both genetic and environmental factors. A stimulating home environment will frequently result in elevated IQ. Parents are often concerned about children's intellectual development, especially when they detect a difference between their child and another child of similar age. In general there is no reason for concern because individual variations exist in the timing of cognitive development. Furthermore, sudden changes, or "spurts" occur at around age six, and then again around age ten. After age eleven spurts become less frequent, and intellectual development follows a more stable pattern. While the average IQ score of children in the United States is approximately 100, it is important to keep in mind that intelligence test scores may be influenced by factors such as a child's physical health, emotional well being, home environment, family dynamics, and educational experiences. Children who consistently score low on IQ tests should receive professional attention from psychologists, educators and pediatricians. Similarly, children whose IQ scores are well above average (at least 130) may need advanced educational opportunities.

Is there a relationship between intelligence and creativity? While an average level of intellectual functioning is necessary for creative endeavors, there are many highly intelligent individuals who lack creativity. Creative people are often unusually productive, independent, nonconformists, unconventional, flexible, inquisitive, and will apply novel solutions to problems. Parents and educators can play a central role in engendering creativity in children. This can be accomplished by having children answer open-ended questions, write essays, formulate opinions, express critical thinking, appreciate music, dance, sculpture and graphic arts, engage in culinary experiences, group discussions and problem solving (groupthink) activities.

In a manner parallel to their marked intellectual development in middle childhood, children's language skills also undergo noticeable changes. These changes not only include grammar, vocabulary and pragmatics (the practical social side of language), but also *metalinguistic awareness*, which is the ability to reflect upon language as an organized system of communication. Exposure to continued formal educational experiences, and reinforcement of correct speaking and writing skills by teachers and parents greatly contribute to these positive changes. The opportunity to communicate in a variety of settings with people of different age groups, and the reward value of being understood provide added motivation for proper language usage. Many children continue to become proficient in more than one language in middle childhood. Allowing children exposure to more than one language at a very early age will greatly facilitate the language learning process. The older children become, the more difficult the acquisition of a second or third language becomes. It is wise to encourage children to develop multilingual skills. Speaking more than one language is very advantageous in our multicultural world.

Moral development is another hallmark of this age bracket. It is predicated on a certain level of intellectual prowess. Psychologist, Lawrence Kohlberg proposed that there are several stages of moral development (Kohlberg, 1981, 1984). Children between the ages of seven and ten operate on the *preconventional level*. At this level children judge morality on the consequences of their behavior. Behavior, which satisfies one's needs, and is not followed by punishment is considered morally appropriate. During middle childhood children begin to reason on a morally more advanced level. This is the *conventional level*. At this level "good" and "bad" behavior are judged by conventional moral standards set by society, or units within the society, such as the family or a religious order. Acting in a way which would make someone else feel good, is also considered important. Sympathy, and complying with the moral behavioral expectations of those around us is also emblematic of this stage. As moral development gradually crystallizes in middle childhood, parental modeling and intervention in this respect is especially important. Most children will readily accept logical explanations of correct moral decisions and conduct. The use of specific and concrete illustrative examples will simplify some of the abstract concepts as we teach children morality.

SECTION 1.10:
SOCIAL AND EMOTIONAL DEVELOPMENT
IN MIDDLE CHILDHOOD

The following topics are discussed in this section:
The influence of the school environment on social
development
Self-knowledge and social cognition
The effect of broken family life and divorce on children
Current knowledge related to lesbian and gay parents

School attendance plays a very significant part in children's lives. The challenges of educational achievement familiarizes children with concepts such as competition, sustained sense of responsibility, goal setting, organization, and time management. The school is also a forum for continued social interactions with peers and adults. The use of respectful manners and pragmatically suitable language are needed when communicating with teachers and other school personnel. Appropriate social skills are essential in order to be accepted by peer groups. Coaches in competitive games also expect correct sportsmanship behaviors. Successful performance in academics, sports, and social activities is closely tied to pride and healthy self-esteem development. Proud and self-confident children will be open to face the challenges for further achievement, and will enjoy school. Some children have special interests and talents, such as playing a musical instrument, dancing, acting, or drawing, which need to be developed after school hours. Parents should recognize and reward children's efforts and positive results. Rewards need not be material or excessive. A kind word, a hug with a smile, or a brief acknowledgement will suffice. Outstanding achievements may merit higher rewards.

In middle childhood children begin to develop self-knowledge related to their intellectual and physical strengths and weaknesses. For example, they may realize that subjects in the areas of mathematics and science are easier for them than language and social studies.

It is important for parents and teachers to encourage children to try their best, but not to admonish them for less than perfect achievement. Some children may need to be taught effective study skills, and may need extra tutoring sessions to prevent failure. Teachers and parents should monitor children's academic progress on a consistent basis. It is advisable for parents to regularly review homework assignments, test results, and report cards. Close contact with teachers is recommended when problems are suspected. Academic weaknesses should be discovered as early as possible, and supportive measures should be provided on a timely manner. When children fall behind in their schoolwork despite honest effort, their achievement motivation often declines. A sense of failure will have negative emotional consequences. The need for parental vigilance in this respect must be emphasized. As we mentioned earlier in this section, authoritative parenting which involves clear limit setting, avoidance of harsh and unreasonable punishment, consistent close involvement with children's lives, love and care, produce youngsters with a generally healthy emotional development, including high self-esteem and a positive self-concept.

In middle childhood children develop a more profound understanding of the relationship between themselves and others. This is called *social cognition*. They begin to appreciate other persons' points of view, and realize that there may be more than "one side to a coin" (Selman, 1980). This kind of cognitive flexibility is essential for critical thinking, creativity, debating, problem solving, and in many other academic and social situations. Social cognition also facilitates the emotional understanding of others, such as the ability to empathize. Children at this stage of development begin to understand some of their personality traits, such as shy, ambitious, friendly, helpful, lazy, and so on. They tend to establish friendships with peers who are similar to their personality, and who enjoy similar activities. The ability to regulate their emotions also increases, as they begin to appreciate the effects that their emotional behavior have on others in their social circles. Frequent hostile expression of anger, for example, may result in social non-acceptance. Some children may require social skills training. Here again, parents need to be vigilant. Children with low self-image may be excessively shy. Girls may feel that they are "not pretty enough", and therefore cannot socially "compete" with some of their friends. They may therefore feel inhibited in their efforts to socialize with peers. Boys may similarly feel inhibited if their physique prevents them from competing successfully in sport activities. Parental encouragement, and sometimes professional counseling may be necessary to prevent further emotional damage and social isolation.

Divorce rate in the United States is very high. According to the U.S. Bureau of the Census report of the year 2004, approximately one million children each year are exposed to the divorce of their parents (U.S. Bureau of the Census, 2004). Considerable research efforts have been expended to study the psychological effects of divorce on children. Very often children harbor anger toward the parent they perceive as the cause for the breakup of the family. These feelings persist for many years. At times children blame themselves for the divorce because they overhear their parents' arguments about childrearing issues. This, of course, is very hurtful. Parents should make every effort to avoid hostile arguments in the presence of their sons and daughters. In the United States mothers usually gain custody of their children. While some fathers maintain close and consistent contact with their sons and daughters, others become progressively more aloof, especially if they engage in a new relationship, and establish a new family. Such lack of involvement deprives children of a variety of activities and social opportunities. Moreover, children become puzzled, and begin to question their self-worth.

Globally speaking, divorce has a negative effect on both boys and girls. Children often show resentment when their mother becomes romantically involved with a man. This kind of involvement necessarily alters the family dynamics. The role of the new man in the family, including the nature of his disciplinary interventions must be clearly established from the very beginning, especially if he stays over nights, or permanently moves in with the mother and her children. While mutual respect should be established, children should not be expected to address the new person as "daddy". Such misguided expectations normally lead to confusion, non-acceptance, and added resentment. Divorced parents ought not alienate, or deprecate a child's mother or father; on the contrary, every effort should be directed toward the facilitation of children's regular access to, and enjoyment of both parents.

Research results point out that children living in broken families are more at risk for lower self-esteem, emotional lability, substance abuse, marginal school performance, and conduct disorders (Amato, 2006; Hetherington, Bridges, & Insabella, 1998). Children who exhibit serious conduct disorders, persistent oppositional behavior, sudden decline in academic performance, anxiety, or depression, will need professional intervention. Initial consultation with a school psychologist is a convenient starting point. Divorce leads to a decline in the quality of parental care, and to the disorganization of family life. A single parent usually has less time to devote to children. Mothers in general need to work long hours to secure financial viability. A tired parent is less patient and less involved in children's school and social lives. Inconsistent parental supervision and lack of daily structure leaves children with little accountability. It is recommended that single parents should make every effort to procure support from immediate family members, such as sisters, brothers, or grandparents. Close friends and after-school programs may be helpful sources as well. Should parents remain married for the sake of their children? It is usually not a good idea to stay married if father and mother do not get along. This is especially true if there are frequent violent fights at home. Children living in unhappy households suffer negative emotional consequences similar to those of divorced parents (Davies & Cummings, 1998). They are anxious, harboring anger, and often blaming themselves for the discord between their mothers and fathers.

Recent studies have focused on the effects of parents' sexual orientation on their children. How adjusted are children of lesbian and gay parents? Contrary to some popular belief, research results indicate that the psychological adjustment of children of lesbian and gay parents is not different from that of heterosexual parents. It was found by several researchers that children raised by gay or lesbian parents have normal cognitive, emotional and social development (Crowl, Ahn, & Baker, 2008). Furthermore, investigations in this field concluded that homosexual men and lesbian women are capable of maintaining a healthy family environment conducive to childrearing (Wainwright, Russell, & Patterson, 2004). In general, the sexual orientation of children raised by gay or lesbian parents is heterosexual (Patterson, 1992, 2003). More precisely, a review of a number of studies showed that these children have a normal variation in gender identity, gender role behavior, and sexual preferences (Smith, Cowie, & Blades, 2003).

SECTION 1.11:
PHYSICAL DEVELOPMENT IN ADOLESCENCE

The following topics are discussed in this section:
Physical and psychological consequences of puberty
The development of body image
Sexual development

Adolescence is a very special stage of development. Major changes occur during these years. This is a transitional period between childhood and adulthood. *Puberty* marks the onset of the adolescent period. This is a time when children reach reproductive capacity as a result of complex biological mechanisms involving brain structures, hormones and sex organs. A small area, deep inside the brain called the *hypothalamus* regulates sexual behavior. A neighboring part of the brain, the *pituitary gland* contains hormones, which control physical growth and gonadal (ovaries and testes) functioning. The gonads produce *androgens* and *estrogens* (sex hormones). The biological structures, which make reproduction possible, are called *primary sex characteristics*. For girls, these include the ovaries, vagina, uterus, and fallopian tubes. For boys, these structures include the penis, testes, prostate gland, and seminal vesicles. The *secondary sex characteristics* do not involve reproductive structures, however they signal the maturation process; for example facial hair and deepening voice in boys, and breast development in girls. Significant height and weight growth spurts (very rapid growth) are to be expected in adolescence.

The body shapes of both boys and girls become more gender specific. Girls gain more fatty tissue than boys, whereas boys gain more muscle tissue than girls (Rathus, 2006). As a consequence of rapid physical changes, adolescents often become preoccupied with their bodies. This is the time when *body image* (the perception and feelings about one's body) develops. In our society girls are very much concerned about their appearance, and there is much emphasis on slimness. Girls often have more negative body images than boys.

This may be attributable to natural body fat increases in puberty. Dangerous weight reduction diets should be avoided. Attention needs to be paid to proper nutrition at this time. While there is a need for sufficient caloric intake to support body growth, a well balanced diet is important to prevent excessive weight gain.

By age thirteen or fourteen boys are able to ejaculate seminal fluid. In girls *menarche* (the onset of menstruation) begins between the ages of eleven and fourteen, but there are individual variations. The onset of menstruation is influenced by several factors. Healthy nourishment and good general health result in earlier menstruation. Menarche is also related to stress. Girls who have been exposed to prolonged periods of stress are more likely to experience earlier onset of menstruation. This trend has been observed in girls whose family life is hostile and turbulent (Ellis, 2004; Golub, 1992). As children reach adolescence they need to receive some education related to sexual behavior, including protective measures such as the use of condoms to prevent pregnancy and sexually transmitted diseases. Girls need to understand the menstrual cycle and associated hygienic care. Although schools do give such information to students, it is important for parents to reinforce matters related to proper sexual conduct. Boys usually feel more comfortable to have such discussions with their father, and girls will prefer to talk to their mother.

SECTION 1.12:
COGNITIVE DEVELOPMENT IN ADOLESCENCE

The following topics are discussed in this section:
The development of inductive and deductive reasoning
Sex differences in cognitive development
Moral reasoning
Transition from elementary school to junior high school
and high school

According to Jean Piaget girls and boys reach the highest level of cognitive functioning in adolescence. This is the stage of "formal operations". It is characterized by abstract thinking, both *inductive* (from the specific to the general) and *deductive* (from the general to the specific) reasoning, and the ability to form hypotheses, to conceptualize, and to classify ideas and objects in a logical manner. The ability to engage in *critical thinking* (the ability to evaluate evidence and think reflectively) also becomes part of advanced intellectual functioning in adolescence. Metacognition, as it was explained earlier, is the ability to think about one's thinking processes. In adolescence this capacity becomes very useful in schoolwork, as youngsters resort to analytical thinking and multi-layered problem solving.

According to a national study conducted in the year 2000 by the United States Department of Education, in general, girls' academic performance is far superior to that of boys. Boys as a group are less attentive in class, and need to receive remedial education more often than girls (U.S. Department of Education, 2000). There are certain sex differences in cognitive abilities. Researchers found that girls' verbal abilities exceed that of boys'. They are also less likely to develop *dyslexia* (reading disorder) than boys. On the other hand, boys excel in visual-spatial abilities. There are some differences in mathematical ability as well. Cultural expectations may play a part in these differences. In countries such as the United States and Canada where reading is viewed as a feminine activity, girls tend to excel; in countries such as Nigeria and England where reading is perceived as a masculine activity, boys surpass girls. Similar cultural trends hold true for visual-spatial and mathematical skills (Rathus, 2006). There are no conclusive biological (brain organization and hormone levels) research findings related to sex differences in cognition.

Moral development also reaches a higher level in adolescence. Psychologist Lawrence Kohlberg posits that adolescents are able to use the *postconventional level* of moral reasoning (Kohlberg, 1984). In other words, their moral judgments are not necessarily derived from conventional standards, laws, regulations, or authority figures. They may base such judgments on their own conscience, ethics, and personal values. Often, however, adolescents reason at lower levels. Sometimes moral thought and moral behavior are not synchronous.

Education continues to be of paramount importance in adolescence. The school environment changes as one transitions from elementary to middle or junior high school. In elementary school classrooms are smaller and better structured than those in middle schools. There are also more teachers involved in the daily educational programs in junior high schools. The general atmosphere is more impersonal. Furthermore, academic demands increase during these years. Parents and teachers need to be aware of the stresses involved as adolescents try to adjust academically and socially to these new circumstances, in addition to the bodily and psychological changes brought about by puberty.

Transition to high school requires a more independent and focused attitude toward academic work. It is wise to start thinking about career preferences during high school years. Many high schools offer specialized training. Guidance counselors should be consulted if students have special academic or vocational interests. Dropping out of high school can have serious consequences for the future. In today's world high school education is a requirement in the workforce. Difficulty coping with academic demands is a consistent cause for leaving school. Parents are urged to detect such problems early, and to formulate remedial plans jointly with school officials. Students who do well in school may be offered several hours of part time employment per week. Gainful employment helps develop discipline, accountability, and responsibility. Excessively long work hours should be avoided, and primary emphasis on schoolwork needs to be consistently maintained. Communication between parents and teachers continues to be important throughout the years of secondary education.

SECTION 1.13:
SOCIAL AND EMOTIONAL DEVELOPMENT
IN ADOLESCENCE

The following topics are discussed in this section:
The formation of identity
Rebellion and effective parental interventions
Peer interactions and the formation of friendships
Dating and romantic relationships
How to prevent and manage teenage pregnancy
Prevention and intervention related to juvenile delinquency

Adolescence marks an important turning point in people's lives. It is during these formative years when critical decisions are made based on newly crystallized perceptions of who we really are. What are my strengths and weaknesses? What are my values and beliefs? Is religion important to me? What are my political views? Do I have any talents? Do I want to go to college? What are my career preferences? What are some of my personality traits? Am I shy or outgoing? Am I ambitious or lazy? Am I a leader or a follower? Do I have creative abilities? Do people like me? Am I a popular person? Am I happy with my appearance? Do I appeal to the opposite sex? Am I ready for dating and sexual relationships? These, and similar other questions need to be answered at this crucial stage of development. One of the most known psychologists who contributed to our understanding of adolescence is Erik Erikson. He stated that adolescents need to develop *ego identity*. In other words they need to define the meaning of their existence. They need to answer some of the questions listed above. This is not an easy task; consideration of these issues requires self-knowledge and exploration of alternatives. Serious reflection and some experimentation may be needed prior to arriving at definitive conclusions. Choices need to be made either alone or with the support of parents, teachers, or counselors.

Parents need to resort to special skills when dealing with adolescents. Frictions frequently occur during these years of development.

This is an expected and normal phenomenon. Adolescents vie for emancipation from parental control. They require freedom to experience life. They defy parental protection and want to learn from their own mistakes. They want to test their own hypotheses about the substance and mechanisms of life. Parents need to respect this rebellion, and gradually loosen the chains of control. Open communication and mutual trust are essential. As adolescents struggle adjusting to their new level of independence, they need to feel a supportive parental cradle, in case they "fall off a cliff". The road leading to independence has many unexpected curves. Parents and adolescents should try to become friends, and form a partnership in sharing new ideas, plans and experiences. Excessive parental protection is not advisable. Parental guidance is most effective when presented as "recommendations", rather than rules and regulations. Instead of escalating arguments, it is often wise to compromise on minor issues such as curfews, chores and dressing habits. Although this may not always be obvious, most adolescents love and respect their parents. They also tend to remember and follow their advices and words of caution even when not in their presence.

Peer relationships have a very central role in adolescents' social and emotional development. Friendship provides necessary social support, as distance increases between children and their families following the onset of puberty. Meaningful interaction with friends also results in emotional security, healthier self-concept, and some aspects of identity formation. Close ties to "best friends" can be very rewarding. Such friendships may become life long. Boys and girls often spend many hours a week in the company of friends. In general, girls' friendships are more intimate than that of boys. Telephone conversations, text-messaging, and e-mailing become an important part of daily life. Unconditional acceptance, loyalty, intimate self-disclosure, sharing of ideas, mutual understanding, and confidentiality are important elements of friendship. Adolescents most often select friends who are similar to them in many ways. They are usually of the same age, sex and race. Their attitudes about school, sports, future goals, sex and drug use are typically similar (Hartup, 1993).

The experience of dating and romantic relationships is a normal aspect of post-puberty life. Appeal to the opposite sex improves self-image. Relating to the opposite sex is also a learning experience with regard to behavior and interests. Approximately forty-five percent of high school students in the United States engage in sexual relationships. Sexually transmitted diseases is a major problem in the United States. Approximately twenty percent of sexually active adolescents suffer from a sexually transmitted disease. These include genital herpes, gonorrhea, syphilis, chlamydia, or AIDS (Shaffer, 2002). Intensive education related to safe sexual behavior is of utmost importance. Adolescents who have a positive and trusting rapport with their mothers and fathers, usually delay sexual activity, and later practice safe sex (McBride, Paikoff, &Holmbeck, 2003).

Teenage pregnancy is a problematic matter. Why do young girls get pregnant? There are several reasons. Many pregnancies are accidental, resulting from unprotected sex. Approximately 50% of high school girls either refuse or do not know how to use condoms. Young girls often do not know how to resist boys' sexual advances. Sometimes they are drunk or under the influence of recreational drugs as they become sexually involved. Some teenagers fall in love, and believe that getting pregnant will ensure a boy's commitment to them (Rathus, 2006. Most teenagers, who elect not to get an abortion, become single parents. Boys are too young to get married, and are not ready for the emotional and financial responsibilities of fatherhood. Naturally the education of teenage mothers gets interrupted because babies need their time and attention. They often end up living in socially and economically deprived environments, with little family support. Their children suffer as well. They frequently develop emotional and behavioral problems, as well as lower levels of cognitive functioning (Coley & Chase-Lansdale, 1998; Miller et al., 1996). Adolescents who become pregnant have little knowledge about prenatal care. They are in need of a variety of services, such as family planning, nutrition, parenting skills training, and health education. A caring family, and the involvement of the father will result in better psychological adjustment for the growing baby.

What can be done to prevent teenage pregnancies? Sex education in public schools can have an influence. Topics such as sexually transmitted diseases, how to use condoms, the functioning of the reproductive system, how to resist peer pressure related to sexual involvements can stimulate adolescents to think more carefully about the consequences of their romantic adventures. Conscious effort should be made to establish a friendly and mature relationship between parents and their growing children. Rather than having to be fearful, adolescents should feel comfortable talking to their parents about their dating experiences. Mothers and fathers should play an advisory role when discussing falling in love, sexual behavior and the responsibilities associated with pregnancy and raising children. It is also helpful for parents to get to know the girlfriends and boyfriends of their children. In families where the relationship between teenagers and parents are hostile, grandparents, aunts and uncles may be a good source of information and support. Appendix IX lists information about measures that can be taken to support pregnant teenagers. Preventive interventions are also addressed.

Juvenile delinquency denotes behaviors, that are illegal. Infractions range from minor events to serious encounters with the law. Most delinquent acts are committed by boys. Why do some adolescents engage in illegal activities? There seem to be some predispositions to delinquent conduct. These include hyperactivity, aggression, antisocial tendencies in early childhood, and parental separation or divorce (Farrington, 2004; Laird et al., 2005). Immature moral reasoning, peer rejection in childhood, low verbal IQ, no interest in school, low self-esteem, substance abuse, and impulsivity are also associated with delinquency. Living in communities with high crime rates is also conducive to delinquent behavior. The increased opportunity to observe criminal behavior and the related rewards for such activities, may motivate adolescents to engage in such behaviors. The family environment plays a significant role as well. Generally speaking authoritative parenting style results in adolescents who are well adjusted (Maccoby & Martin, 1983). On the other hand authoritarian parents who are aloof, and use frequent harsh punishment with little justification produce anger, rebellion, and tendencies for violence in their children. Overly lenient parents, on the other hand, fail to instill or enforce necessary behavioral limits at home (See chapter 2, section 2 for a description of parenting styles). These children fail to respect the law, and the rights and properties of others.

Studies have shown that the parents of many juvenile delinquents have histories of antisocial or criminal activities (Rowe, Rodgers, & Meseck-Bushey, 1992). Juvenile delinquency can be prevented and treated. Some programs provide training in social and problem-solving skills, and moral reasoning (Gibbs et al., 2009). Other programs have a more systemic approach, involving families, schools and communities (Chamberlain & Reid, 1998). Early childhood intervention programs emphasize preventive measures, including social skills counseling, academic remediation, parenting skills training, and family therapy. See Appendix X for programs aimed at the prevention and treatment of juvenile delinquency.

CHAPTER TWO:

Parents and Children

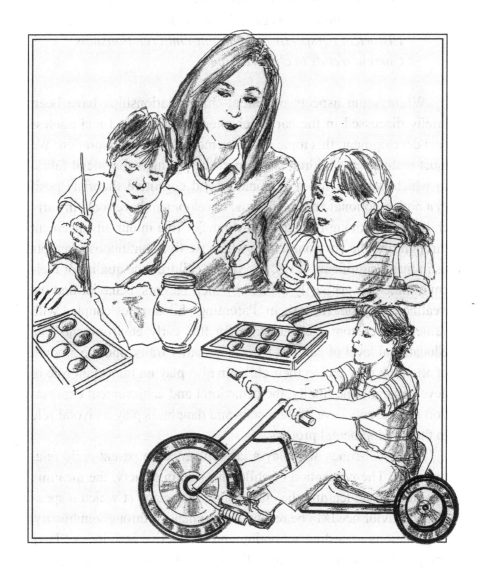

*"Having children makes one
no more a parent than having a
piano makes you a pianist."*
MICHAEL LEVINE

SECTION 2.1:
INTRODUCTION AND HISTORY

The following topics are discussed in this section:
Determining factors related to parenthood
Historical perspectives on parent-child relationships
Current trends in child rearing

While some aspects of parent-child relationships have been briefly discussed in the earlier chapters on childhood and adolescent development, this topic deserves more detailed exploration. We must realize that children are in part the products the social fabric in which we live. Most personality and cognitive theorists posit that both emotional and intellectual development have roots in early childhood. Although genetics play a major role in our advancement through life, the environment in which we live continuously sculpts us in many significant ways. For young children the quality of their environment is primarily defined by their parents' behavior and the treatment they get from them. Parenting philosophies coupled with values and customs set the stage for this early environment. The educational level of parents, their personality traits, and the amount of attention they pay to their children also play an important role in development. And finally, the behavioral and achievement expectation that parents have of their sons and daughters play a pivotal role in the developmental process.

Historical times also play a key influence on parent-child relationships. The perception of children's role in society, the meaning of mature conduct, and the anticipation of the age at which responsible behavior needs to be reached have changed throughout history. Expectations regarding schooling and productive activities of boys and girls have similarly changed throughout times past. In contemporary times in takes longer to "grow up". It is not unusual for teenagers and young adults to pursue their formal education, and to rely on their parents' support until their mid-twenties. Gainful employment often commences only following many years of schooling and training.

This trend, of course, is partially a reflection of our specialized advanced technological and scientific era. But it is also a manifestation of our tolerance and perception of nurturing in our current Western culture. We raise our children in accordance with the needs we ascribe for their success in their future lives.

As we glance back on the annals of history we shockingly realize the changes that paved the way to our present modes of relating to our children. A child's life in ancient Greece and Rome was not much fun. Childhood ended by age seven, or even earlier. At this early age boys were expected to assume adult responsibilities such as engaging in physical productive work. Parents, especially mothers were expected to teach their children basic knowledge related to their culture. Boys were expected to gain formal education, while girls were taught domestic skills and child care management. Children who were not suited for schooling, work or domestic chores were often deserted. Some of them were sold by their fathers and relegated to slavery. Women and children were "owned" by men, who were the supporters and heads of households. Abusive conditions prevailed during the Middle Ages (400-1400 A.D.) as well. Children's needs were rarely considered as important. By age seven they were regarded as "miniature adults", and were expected to conduct themselves accordingly, and to learn skills, mostly agricultural, needed to make a living. Formal education was offered only to the privileged few. Children learned by observing the behavior and lifestyle of their fathers and mothers. As medical knowledge was very primitive during this time in history, many children died at an early age.

During the period of European Renaissance (1400-1600 A.D.) the fate of children was not much better. Little emphasis was paid to the quality of parenting and the needs of children. Not until the end of the Renaissance were children treated as "children". Around this time there emerged noticeable changes in the medical care and parenting methods of young boys and girls. There appeared to be a semblance of sensitivity to their developmental requirements.

We know that our political, social, cultural, and religious origins emerged from European influences. It logically follows then that

85

child rearing in our country was similarly affected by European views. The social atmosphere in Colonial America (1600-1800 A.D.) gave birth to many radical changes in the perception of the nature of children. While parents acted responsibly and with affection toward their sons and daughters, they viewed them as inherently evil. It was the prevailing belief that in order to help children overcome their depraved nature harsh punitive measures must be taken. Children were subjected to severe disciplinary methods and hard labor. Christian doctrine insisted that parents should be obeyed at all times. Play activities were restricted. Religious involvement and moral instruction were strictly enforced. Again, as in previous times, children were expected to assume adult behavior at an early age.

Fundamental changes in family life and parental roles took place around the time of the Industrial Revolution (1800-1860). Agricultural lifestyle and employment of fathers on farms was replaced by factory jobs. This shift in employment opportunities resulted in fathers being separated from their families for considerable time periods. Hence the role of the father as the ultimate disciplinarian was fading away. Mothers became the most influential role models for children. Parenting techniques of ruthless punishment gave way to more explanatory means of socialization and nurturance of children. The writings of the English philosopher, John Locke (1632-1704) were especially dominant in the shaping of people's understanding of child development (Locke, 1699). He emphatically stated that children are born innocent with no experiences of their own. Locke's "tabula rasa" concept holds that we are born with minds resembling a blank slate. Our experiences drawn from the environment in which we are brought up determines our personalities. Therefore the behavior of our parents as role models, the learning environment and opportunities they provide, and the approaches they use as they rear us serve as crucial factors in our ultimate character development as we progress toward adulthood.

Our current attitudes toward parenting and the developmental needs of children are in part attributable to European influences in the nineteenth century. There was a tendency to abandon the perception of children as naturally bad. Rather they were viewed as ignorant and helpless who needed to be taught right from wrong in a supportive, nurturing manner. Harsh punishment was discouraged. Reasonable explanations with rewards for appropriate behaviors were suggested. Early formal childhood education was recommended. Parents were encouraged to enroll their kids in nursery schools and kindergartens.

Significant changes took place in the 20th century with regard to child rearing. These changes were in many ways related to the teachings of professionals whose interest was in child development. The writings of psychoanalysts such as Sigmund Freud, Carl Jung, Alfred Adler, Karen Horney, and Erik Erikson emphasized the importance of supportive parental care and consistent attention to the needs of children in their formative years. As psychology became a recognized scientific discipline, experimentally proven behavioral principles were recommended to parents as effective methods for modifying their children's behavior. Psychologists advocated the application of rewards for desired behaviors, and informed caretakers about the negative effects of severe punishment. While mothers were considered to be the primary nurturers, fathers were advised to participate in childcare as much as time allowed. The introduction of child labor laws, and mandatory public education put an end to the widespread exploitation of children on farms and factories. As a result of the Women's Movement towards social equality coupled with the need for additional income, the structure of family life underwent significant alterations. As women joined the workforce and had less time for domestic responsibilities, men became more involved in parenting and household tasks. Given the difficult economic conditions of our time and the desire of women to maintain a significant foothold in the job market, this trend of changed gender roles in families has been continuing to present days. Furthermore, the need for higher education and specialized training for employment in our generation necessitates children to depend on parental support for an extended period of time before achieving financial independence.

SECTION 2.2:
APPROACHES TO CHILD REARING: GENERAL CONCEPTS

The following topics are discussed in this section:
A review of theories related to child rearing
A description of effective parenting
An examination of behavior modification techniques

As there is no universal prescription for child rearing techniques, the manner in which we bring up our children in a very personal undertaking. As we have learned in the previous section, parenting practices are much influenced by personal factors such as education, philosophy, childhood memories and a variety of expectations. Religion, tradition and societal customs are also important determinants. In our modern times behavioral scientists have done much research on effective parenting. Results of such studies have been infused into the awareness of the general population in developed societies. Insofar as causation in psychology is quite multifaceted, there are numerous theoretical perspectives on effective parenting skills. Prior to the 20th century children were expected to abide by parental standards and follow instructions in an unquestionable manner. The family atmosphere was militaristic, and rules of the house were inflexible. In today's world there is more flexibility between parents and children. In most households there is a give-and-take process in the communication of standards of behavior and parental expectations. Children are offered explanations for the rationale behind morality and proper social conduct. They are allowed to question and opinionate on the value system imposed upon them.

Family systems theory explains the dynamics which govern communication, decision making, goal setting, and rules of demeanor within the family unit. This dynamic is bi-directional; this means that the behavior of family members can influence one another. Environmental factors such as our neighborhoods, and cities as well as and the individual's interaction with the social surroundings and access to social programs have much bearing on development. The *family ecological theory* explains the environmental effects on child rearing and on the operation of the family unit (Berk, 2010). Learning theory describes the effects of rewards and punishments on behavior, and the implementation of behavior modification techniques. Observational learning is the domain of *social learning theory*. This involves behaviors which arise as a result of observation and imitation of others (Nevid, 2013). The development of problem-solving skills, and information processing has been explored by cognitive theorists such as Jean Piaget, and later by other cognitive scientists (Reed, 1997). Finally, the *sociocultural theory* of the Russian psychologist, Lev Vygotsky talks about how interactions with parents and other adults can stimulate the intellectual development of children (Vygotsky, 1978). Delving into the details of these developmental theories is outside the scope of this book. Interested readers may turn to the reference section of this book for information about further reading on such topics.

Effective parenting is a skillful process. Some of us are more adept than others. Sensitivity, patience, nurturance, and teaching are essential elements of child rearing. Close familiarity with children's emotionality, sensitivities, strengths and weaknesses are equally important. Authoritarian parenting styles where excessive control is employed should be avoided. Parental intimidation fosters emotional maladjustment and inhibits creativity and motivation. Research in this area indicates that the *authoritative style* of parenting is the preferred one. This approach to parenting is characterized by reasoning, explaining, and demonstrating in the process of socializing children. While parents exercise reasonable control and use mild punitive measures when the need arises, a democratic family atmosphere is preserved. Children are allowed to question and comment on parental values and regulations. This parenting style is conducive to the development of autonomy, self-reliance, and intellectual growth in youngsters (Bigner, 2010).

Some parents are "eager teachers", in their attempts to push their sons and daughters to the limit. We need to be mindful of the fact that children's biological readiness for learning is variable. The physical and psychological maturational process is a subjective phenomenon. Hence good judgment must be exercised in setting expectations. Children's learning ability is predicated on their neurological development. Insisting on teaching children skills, which they are not ready to acquire results in frustration and even aversion to future learning. The patient and gradual approach to training bears fruit: children need to experience success in order to enjoy the learning process, and to sustain motivation and curiosity.

What is it that parents teach their young? Looking at our animal ancestry can provide a quick answer. What do birds teach their chicks? They model flying techniques, and perhaps fishing as a way to procure food. What do tigers teach their cubs? They teach them how to find and pursue potential prey in a stealthy manner. They teach them methods of capturing and killing their victim. These are skills necessary for survival. As we look at the animal kingdom and evolution this tendency of learning survival skills from parents has been a recurring phenomenon in most if not all species. We humans have been adhering to the exact same evolutionary tradition. Historically we have been teaching our children skills required for survival. Parents draw upon their experiences and wisdom as they shape their children to acquire the competencies needed for successful continued existence in the world into which they were born. This includes proper social behavior, as well as specific abilities to facilitate future employment opportunities. In the early years of civilization parents, especially mothers, had a significant and in many ways exclusive role in preparing their kids for adulthood. Over the centuries of progressive technological and scientific expansions and with the advent of mandated formal education in modern civilized societies, parents became facilitators rather than teachers. The acquisition of both basic and advanced academic and technical knowledge takes place in schools, training centers and universities. However, the fundamental skills related to human relations and moral behaviors are still learned at home. Generational customs, traditions and values are also embedded in the home environment.

The process of learning anything involves motivation and active effort. Both psychological and physiological changes occur as we learn. While some learning experiences are inherently rewarding, such as learning how to use language at a young age, others may cause discomfort, leading to resistance; toilet training of toddlers is an example. The socialization process of children frequently generates resistance. Why is this the case? Two reasons pop in mind: children have a limited appreciation for the ramifications of impolite or socially frowned upon behaviors. Also, it is generally easier to engage in instinctive and more primitive behaviors, than follow refined social customs. Historical documents show us that parents have been resorting to a variety of disciplinary measures in their attempts to counteract children's resistance to socialization efforts. The nature of these corrective measures have in a large part been associated with prevailing perceptions of the role of children in society, and the definition of parent-child relationships. As described above, in earlier periods severe corporal punishments were customary. With the passage of time children were gradually treated in a more humane manner. As psychology evolved into an organized field of study, much research was devoted to establish effective means for behavior modification.

Although modern industrialized countries do offer formal parent education classes, most prospective mothers and fathers do not take advantage of such services, unless mandated by courts of law, such as in cases of child abuse. College educated people who take courses in psychology may get some exposure to the principles of proper parenting. Some parents who find their children difficult to manage may resort to the guidance of mental health professionals. The fact of the matter is that the great majority of adults use their instincts, memories of their own upbringing, life experiences, and common sense as they rear their children. Societal strictures such as laws related to child labor and abusive punitive measures also influence parent-child relationships. In general, what are our goals as we discipline our children? Preparation for adulthood is the common purpose. Inculcation of the rules and values governing the existing social structure is essential. Of equal importance is the appropriate use of *emotional regulation*. This includes sharpening one's ability to delay gratification, and to control impulsive behavior. Children need to learn to use reasoned judgment before acting.

Numerous psychology books and self-help manuals have been published on the topic of *behavior modification*. The essential strategies for changing children's behavior are as follows: 1) Both positive and negative behaviors require parental attention and recognition. Unfortunately in most households unwanted behaviors draw frequent attention, while proper behaviors are treated as "expected", with no recognition offered. Hence good behavior is not reinforced. 2) As indicated above, children's developmental readiness must be taken into account prior to setting expectations. 3) Reasons for rules need to be explained in an age-appropriate language. Where possible, some room should be offered for negotiation. 4) Showering children with too many rules should be avoided. 5) When rewards or punishments are promised, these should be delivered in a timely and consistent manner. Heed needs to be taken about the effectiveness of rewards and punishments. This requires close knowledge of children's likes and dislikes. 6) Overindulgence for ordinary achievement and expected behaviors should be minimized; in the same vein, excessive punishments for minor infractions are often harmful. 7) Negative comments and criticisms should be directed at *actions* rather than at the person who committed the improper behavior. For example, instead of saying: "You are a cruel boy because you hit your little sister", it is preferable to say, "Hitting your little sister is a cruel thing to do". This manner of communication prevents damage to children's self image. 8) Parents ought not engage in behaviors which contradict the "rules of the house". For example, if children are forbidden to use abusive language, parents should refrain from using foul words as well. Children are very observant; unintentionally modeled behaviors are frequently imitated. 9) When punishment is meted out a detailed explanation should be offered describing the reasons for the punitive measures taken. It is important for children not to equate punishment with withdrawal of love. Excessive and misunderstood punishment may backfire in the form of rebellion. 10) In families with multiple children each child's individuality, such as preferences for activities, personality traits, strengths and weaknesses must be recognized and respected. "Quality time" must be spent which each child separately, as well as jointly. This will facilitate a healthy progression toward the establishment of a positive self-esteem. Admonishments in the form of comparing one child's behavior or accomplishment to another are to be avoided. Competition for achievement and associated parental rewards should also be discouraged.

SECTION 2.3:
PARENTAL CARE OF INFANTS AND TODDLERS

The following topics are discussed in this section:
Parenting skills and sensitivities needed in the care of infants and toddlers
Psychological issues related to breast-feeding
The facilitation of secure attachment
Promoting a sense of autonomy in toddlers

This early developmental stage is of crucial importance. Infancy and toddlerhood includes the first three years of life following birth. The skills acquired at this time set the stage for further abilities later in life. These include both physical and psychological functions such as motor coordination needed for walking and manual dexterity, and the beginning of receptive and expressive capacities, which lay the foundations for language development. Parental sensitivity and vigilance are essential at this time. The facilitation of a trustful relationship between infants and caretakers is crucial. From an infant's perspective parents are the representatives of the world at large. In the opinion of many child psychologists an infant's initial impressions of the quality of parental care have a significant bearing on adult *social perceptions.* Consistent and emotionally warm care promotes social cooperation in later years. Unpredictable presence of caretakers in times of need and aloof parental attitudes foster suspicion and mistrust in people in later adult interpersonal relationships. In view of the fact that children are basically helpless in their early months after birth, and are limited in their abilities to express their needs, parental alertness and anticipation of their infant's requirements cannot be overstated.

Assuring optimal physical and psychological development requires a nutritious and regular feeding schedule, as well as medical monitoring when needed. Timely information about immunizations against diseases such as polio, measles, mumps, and diphtheria must be obtained from pediatricians. Periodic visits to pediatricians are recommended in order to ascertain that major developmental landmarks have been met by infants. Early detection of physical or psychological abnormalities allow for timely rehabilitative efforts. Many years ago breast-feeding was the only way to nourish infants. As baby formulas were developed, there were choices to be made regarding the feeding process. As there are some psychological ramifications to breast-feeding, it is advisable that choices related to feeding of infants should be discussed by both parents. Early psychoanalysts held that breast-feeding is crucial in the psychological bonding process between mother and child. It has been further suggested that this bonding is necessary for proper psychological adjustment later in life. While there is no solid scientific evidence to prove the relationship between breast-fed babies and the quality of their adjustment later in life, many developmental specialists still tend to promote the natural choice, especially in the early weeks following birth.

Interestingly, there is another consideration with regard to feeding. In my years of clinical practice as I collaborated with pediatricians, pediatric nurses and psychologists, it has come to my attention that some men experience stressful reactions as their wives engage in breast-feeding. They feel that the baby has become the primary focus of their wife's attention and affection. Open and honest communication between husband and wife is helpful in the prevention of feelings of jealousy on the part of the husband. Husbands should be actively involved in all aspects of childcare. While it is often easy for wives to be fully enveloped in the new role of "mother", they should make every effort to spend sufficient time with their husbands. Undeniably infants require much time and attention. Let us not forget however that adults need attention as well. Parents must assure that their marital bond should remain solid. Therefore quality private time must be devoted for the maintenance of a happy marriage. In turn, happy marriages pave the way for appropriate childcare, and well-adjusted children.

Parents often wonder when to initiate weaning. Some authorities claim that infants may be offered solid foods as early as fourteen weeks after birth, while others recommend weaning between six to eight months of age. Tradition oriented parents prefer home cooked soft meals for their infants; others resort to commercially prepared baby foods. Both approaches work well as long as the essential nutrients are provided. Proper dietary needs of infants may be obtained from pediatric nurses and dieticians.

In general it is wise to provide structure and consistent care to infants. In the early months of life this means responding in a timely manner to infants' discomfort, anticipating their needs and feeding at regular intervals. The aim is to establish a trustworthy relationship between infants and caretakers. Maintaining eye contact while holding and feeding infants further supports the bonding process. Regular morning and afternoon nap times should also be introduced to toddlers. At night the bedtime hour should also be regulated. It is not uncommon for toddlers to resist going to bed. Sleep resistance may be associated with fear of scary dreams, fear of darkness, or fear of being left alone. A newly experienced sense of independence may contribute to this bedtime-related negativism. A brief pleasant story or lullaby and a small dim light bulb in the toddler's room often allay sleep-related anxieties. Bedtime hours should not be negotiable; they need to be firmly established and routinized by parents. Usually over a short time period toddlers internalize these patterns without much parental intervention. Continued structure and affectionate caring should be maintained throughout the period of infancy and toddlerhood.

Parents need to be vigilant and sensitive to the infant's ever changing developmental needs. Supportive attention should be paid to toddlers' attempts to engage in gradually more advanced tasks. It is generally unwise for parents to "rush" the developmental progress of toddlers. It is unnecessary to utilize training walkers and sophisticated play equipments in an attempt to "help" infants muster new motor or mental tasks. If given a reasonably stimulating home environment including simple toys, verbal and non-verbal communication, healthy toddlers respond well to nature's pathways. Providing positive feedback and encouragement by means of smiling, caressing, holding or talking to infants by both parents and other caretakers is advisable. Harsh criticisms and punishments should be avoided at this stage.

Every effort should be made to foster an environment where toddlers should feel securely attached to their caretakers. Secure attachment is achieved as toddlers experience that their nutritional and comfort needs are met in a timely and predictable manner. Consistent expression of love, physical closeness, frequent verbal interaction and eye contact are also necessary for optimal bonding. Securely attached toddlers ordinarily are more adventurous, and less fearful in unfamiliar situations, and in the presence of strangers. As they grow up, securely attached toddlers have an easier time forming new social contacts, friendships, and trusting intimate relationships.

Attempts to establish a sense of autonomy is a major hallmark of early development. This endeavor on the part of toddlers is often accompanied by tensions between them and their parents. As this struggle for independence involves the beginnings of self-definition and self-regulation including the setting of personal boundaries between the self of toddlers and others, negativistic behaviors are to be expected. The will of toddlers may at times be in opposition to parental demands. Parents need to manage such power struggles with patience and tact. While reasonable parental guidance and safety measures must be in place, toddles need to be allowed sufficient space to exercise their efforts toward *autonomy*. Hence some give-and-take and compromise are advisable in this process. Toddlers need to feel that they are able to separate themselves from their parents, and that they are able to accomplish simple tasks in an independent fashion and according to their own time schedule.

Strict parental control and punishments should be avoided at this juncture. Proper toilet training procedures are especially important as toddlers vie for self-sufficiency. Parental anxieties and intense anticipations related to toilet training should not be conveyed to toddlers. Rather, toddlers need gentle and patient guidance as they go through this important transition. They need to feel competent in this respect to meet parental expectations independently, in accordance with their chronological readiness. It is a big mistake on the part of parents to rush the toilet training process, or to shame and punish toddlers when accidental soiling occurs. Patience, recognition of toddlers' efforts to comply, and positive reinforcement most often result in successful and psychologically healthy toilet training.

As kids continue to enjoy their newly discovered self-governing capacities, they will want to satisfy their curiosities by engaging in a host of *exploratory behaviors*, such as reaching for a variety of objects around the house, or crawling behind curtains or pieces of furniture. Again, while parents need to be mindful about safety concerns, excessive stricture and overprotection should be avoided. Toddlers need reasonable freedom in order for them to feel a sense of accomplishment as they attempt to discover and understand their environment. Continued success in these initial activities, accompanied by parental reassurance, will lead to motivation for further learning.

SECTION 2.4:
PARENTING PRACTICES FOR PRESCHOOLERS

The following topics are discussed in this section:
The psychological characteristics and needs of young
children
Parenting skills required for guiding preschool children
The socialization of preschoolers
Development of gender identity
Effective disciplining techniques
The role of parents in children's intellectual development

In this section the discussion will focus on children between the ages of three and six. The quest for autonomy clearly continues in this age bracket. Parallel to the biological development of the nervous system children's motor and cognitive capacities undergo noticeable changes. Increased expressive and receptive abilities and a more advanced vocabulary allows for improved communication. Personality traits also become more differentiated. At this stage children insist on getting certain privileges and attempt engaging in certain activities despite their parents' disapproval. As children test the limits of their freedom, conflicts may arise in families. Early childhood is marked by a number of developmental landmarks. As compared to toddlers, there is a slower rate of physical growth in the preschool years. However gross motor skills such as running and handling objects are quite well developed. Children at this age are curious, and are willing to explore, experiment, and learn. It is wise for parents to provide ample opportunities for learning at this phase of life. Access to a variety of toys, visits to museums, zoos, parks, movies, and recreation areas is recommended. Children should be encouraged to ask questions and be given answers at the level appropriate for their cognitive development.

Opportunities for social experiences should also be offered. It is good practice to introduce children to others of the same age, and to plan joint activities, such as trips to nearby amusement parks.

Children greatly benefit from such social encounters, including the learning of basic social skills such as sharing of toys and taking turns in games and rides. Children's communication skills also improve as they try to convey information and converse with their peers. Parental recognition and affirmation of children's accomplishments in all areas is essential to promote further motivation in the learning process. Parental guidance is needed in helping children appreciate *gender identity* and become cognizant of behaviors typical of both sexes. Sex-role development begins soon after birth. Parents are the facilitators in this process. They assign a gender appropriate name to the child and dress him or her in clothes and colors which conform to gender related cultural customs. The learning of sex-appropriate behaviors is ordinarily initiated in the family system, as children observe their parents' conduct and activities around the house. As preschoolers begin to interact with their peers, the mode of functioning of same-sex children further defines and reinforces sex appropriate behaviors.

Traditional gender roles have undergone significant alterations in industrial societies. As women gradually joined the workforce and have become breadwinners in the past several decades, house chores and child rearing activities are often shared in married couples. Both men and women spend time in the kitchen, and attend to their infants' needs. In preparation for the realities of life, it is wise for parents to raise their children in the spirit of flexible sex role concepts. Children's curiosities branch out in all directions, including seeking information about sexual issues. It is common for preschoolers to inquire about pregnancy and childbirth. This is especially true when their mother becomes pregnant and a baby is expected to be born. It is psychologically healthy for children to be familiar with the "facts of life". Hence questions related to such topics should be addressed in an emotionally mature and satisfying manner, using language suitable for preschoolers' limited intellectual capacities. Most public libraries hold books on topics of pregnancy and childbirth suitable for children. Appendix XIX lists recommended literature for this purpose.

Family members should refrain from ridiculing and teasing children as they struggle with the socialization and sex-role acquisition process. Sarcastic and humiliating remarks may generate shame, and can have an inhibitory effect on the developmental course. Conflicting messages should not be used. For example if a child is forbidden to use foul language, parents need to refrain from using profanities as well. We need to be mindful of the fact that children are keen listeners and observers. They readily emulate adult behaviors. The "rules of the house" and other regulations need to be explained in a logical and comprehensible manner. As children understand the reasons for the "do's and don'ts", compliance usually improves. Sometimes children try to negotiate rules. It is good practice to identify the *negotiable and non-negotiable rules*, and to give reasons for each. It is poor practice to say the following: "You must go to bed at eight o'clock, because I said so...and remember, I am your mother". Ordinarily the non-negotiable rules involve safety, health, and good citizenship. The consequences associated with the violation of non-negotiable rules should be spelled out. Children need to be told that punishment is not synonymous with the withdrawal of love. In fact punishment should be viewed as a constructive measure to protect children and teach them right from wrong. While punitive actions should be meted out consistently and immediately following the wrongful act, they should not be excessively harsh. Corporal punishment should be avoided. *Withdrawal of favored privileges* or *time out* of preferred activities usually work well. The severity of punishment should never be out of proportion with the level of wrongful behavior. Very severe and capricious punitive methods can backfire. Children may become overly intimidated, inhibited, withdrawn or rebellious. Negotiable rules, on the other hand, can prompt children to think and reason as they attempt to solve problems, resolve conflicts, and protect their own interests. For example, a boy may refuse to share his toy with his brother for a "good reason", such as having a previous experience when his toy was returned to him in a broken condition. Parents are urged to listen patiently to children's logic, and to respond in a just manner. Reasoning with young children and ushering them in the right direction as they interact with family members, other adults and peers can be a challenging task.

As a general rule, in order to prevent insulting a child and putting him or her on the defensive it is prudent to separate a child's personality from the behaviors which need modification. For example, it is unwise to say the following: "Hitting your sister shows me that you are a nasty and mean child". The preferred way is: "I am very angry to learn that you hit your sister and caused her to cry". This latter method reduces the chances for defensive behavior, and preserves a child's healthy self-esteem. It is counterproductive to instill guilt feeling to children. Experiencing guilt invokes disturbing emotions, which interfere with logical thinking. In the same vein, recognition of a positive achievement should be directed at the event itself rather than at the child. This approach prevents the formation of an "inflated ego". For example, it is proper to say: "It makes me happy to see that you are helping your grandmother drying the dishes." While it is appropriate to praise children periodically, it is not recommended to use remarks such as this one too frequently: "I see you are a wonderful and courteous child as you are helping your grandmother drying the dishes." It is commonplace to see parents admonishing children for their misbehavior, without guiding them toward the correct alternative. Take for example, the following comment: "Stop hitting and cursing at your younger brother!" A preferred alternative is: "If you are angry with your younger brother, tell him why you are angry, and what you expect of him...hitting him is inappropriate!"

Preschoolers need to be socialized. This significant process prepares children for a healthy adjustment to the social and cultural milieu in which they conduct their daily life. This includes skills related to initiating friendships, respecting the rights of others, the ability to *empathize* (to show awareness of other people's feelings), and to be inclined to help others when such need arises. Hostile aggression and impulsiveness need to be discouraged. Repeatedly teaching children to wait and think before they act is important. Training them to think in terms of consequences is equally vital. Properly socialized children become respectable citizens later in life.

Given that children at this age tend to be selfish and self-centered, the learning of "civilized" comportment and the exhibition of prosocial behaviors are difficult tasks to master. Consistent parental reminders and frequently modeled desirable ways of behaving are beneficial in helping along the road to socialization.

In order to help children in their intellectual development, parents need to be familiar with the nature of children's cognitive capacities in this age bracket. This information is reviewed in Chapter One of this book. Effective communication with eye contact between parents and children is essential. Patient listening to questions, even if they become repetitious, is helpful. Explaining meanings of words, and associating words with objects, events, feelings, and simple concepts is equally useful. Involving children in conversations stimulates listening skills and the proper timing and formulation of responses. Urging children to recount the day's events is especially valuable. In doing so, children learn to think retrospectively, and organize their thoughts in a sequentially sound fashion. Asking preschoolers to talk about upcoming activities promotes the usage and understanding of the future tense, and the cognitive ordering of future concepts. Attention should be paid to correct sentence structure and grammatical usage, including the proper application of irregular verbs. Selected books, toys and games also stimulate cognitive development.

SECTION 2.5:
PARENTING IN THE MIDDLE CHILDHOOD YEARS

The following topics are discussed in this section:
Children's adjustment to school academically and socially
The role of parents in children's academic achievement and
social acceptance
Teaching children to appreciate the value of money
The development of self-image and self-esteem in middle
childhood

Great challenges await parents of children between six years of age and puberty. The expectations of parents and children of each other dramatically change. Children need increasingly more psychological space to grow, and in turn they need to convince parents that they are able to put new freedoms to safe and constructive use. As biological growth continues, new cognitive and psychosocial abilities unfold. The need for responsible behavior emerges as children enter the public or private school system. Children need to get adjusted to life outside the protective home environment. Getting used to the regular practice of conventional social skills and socialized behaviors learned during the preschool years becomes increasingly important. Periodic parental reminders and monitoring of appropriate behaviors is advisable.

As children become aware of the new social and academic expectations placed upon them, their sense of self undergoes a variety of changes as well. As they attempt to accomplish the daily academic tasks and associated social necessities, they gradually become aware of their strengths and weaknesses. Their self-concept is also influenced by the feedback they receive from their teachers and peers. Repeated academic and social successes bolster a healthy self-esteem. However they also may become vulnerable to psychological bruises as they compare their school performance to that of their classmates. Their perceived inferior classroom work may become a cause for anxiety. Insufficient social acceptance by peers may become a source of disappointment. Parental vigilance and sensitivity to the possibility of such problems is of great importance. A friendly and tolerant home atmosphere provides a safe haven for children following the trials during the hours spent in school. It is wise for parents to encourage boys and girls to honestly relate at home the day's academic and social events, which had taken place in school. Both positive and negative experiences should be addressed. Reinforcement for successful performance should be given; solutions for hurtful events should be sought. It is highly recommended that parents should keep in touch with teachers. Regular contact including participation in parent-teacher conferences provides parents with first hand information about their son's and daughter's classroom behavior and scholastic progress. Furthermore, teachers get a sense of the support pupils receive at home. Thus they can readily advise parents how to assist in correcting particular academic or social difficulties children may experience in school. Some children experience below average academic progress despite long hours of honest effort doing their work. This pattern of difficulty may be attributable to a learning impediment or an emotional disturbance. Early diagnosis by a child psychologist and pediatric neurologist is crucial. Special educational assistance, medication and psychotherapy may be needed in some cases. The necessity for parental attention and support as children enter school cannot be overstated. The ultimate aim is to assure that children should readily accept intellectually and emotionally the new learning environment, and that they should *want* to go to school.

In order to effectuate satisfactory school performance it behooves parents to introduce new *non-negotiable* regulations at home. The purpose of these rules should be to instill regularities with regard to school-related responsibilities, and to prioritize daily activities. Upon arriving home from school, it is a good idea to let children enjoy a small snack, and rest for about an hour. Immediately following this rest period homework is to be started. Children should be responsible for knowing the nature of the assigned homework. They should make every attempt to do their homework assignment independently in a neat and organized manner. Upon conscientiously completing their assignment parents should review their work, and opinionate on neatness, organization and correctness of the written material. When needed, parents should offer guidance in order to arrive at correct answers. If parents feel that a child's work is sloppy, or that insufficient effort has been demonstrated, the child should be required to redo the assignment in a careful manner. It is not unusual for children to initially have to repeat doing assignments several times until they realize the quality of work expected of them by teachers and parents. Given that young children's attention span is quite short, it is advisable to allow them brief rest periods in the course of homework preparation. If parents are not in a position to help children with their homework, perhaps as a result of long work hours, limited education, or insufficient familiarity with the English language, another qualified relative or friend should be appointed for this purpose. Participation in after-school programs is another alternative.

Rules at home should address the importance of doing homework daily at regularly designated times in a quiet room with no distractions. Play activities are to be predicated on successful completion of homework assignments. Keeping in mind that school-age children need about ten hours of sleep, bedtime must be respected. Sleepy and tired children cannot keep up with the rigors of schoolwork. Extracurricular involvements such as sports, religious instruction, dancing and music lessons should not interfere with academic work. Parents need to exercise good judgment when they sign up their sons and daughters for such activities. Children have limited time and energy; they also need rest and time for recreation!

Now a few words about money. As children enter school and spend extended time periods away from home, it is a good idea to introduce them to the *use of money*, as well as the *functional value* and *symbolic meaning* that money represents. As children learn to identify change (pennies, nickels, dimes and quarters) parents can give them a small amount of pocket money to purchase snacks in a school cafeteria. As they make their purchases, and as they see their peers buying various items, they will soon learn that the more money they have, the more things they can buy. They may ask parents to increase their daily allowance. This provides a good opportunity for parents to discuss the work and energy that is involved in earning money.

Given the fact that young children's conceptual understanding is narrow, resorting to concrete methods of instruction is quite useful. It is advisable to assign children a few simple house chores, such as helping folding laundry, drying dishes, setting the dinner table, or dusting furniture. Upon satisfactory completion of such chores, a small amount of money may be earned. This simple practice is a worthy educational tool. Children quickly discover that "money does not grow on trees". They learn to associate the expenditure of work energy with the accumulation of money. The advantages of saving money can also be introduced at this time. Here a piggybank can serve a good purpose. Children will soon realize that as funds accumulate they will be able to purchase items that they could not afford earlier. Borrowing money from others, or lending should be discouraged. The appreciation of basic economics in childhood sets the stage for prudent monetary decisions in later adult life.

As children grow and develop, their *self-image* and *self-esteem* changes. These psychological changes are influenced by a variety of factors. The ability to live up to *increased responsibilities* as expected by parents is one such determinant. So is the ability to make sound decisions independently. For instance, parents may expect children to wake up in the morning on time in order not to be late to school. Thus boys and girls will learn to set the alarm clock daily before going to bed. Parents may expect children to dress appropriately for school, keeping weather conditions in mind. Children in turn may listen to weather reports, and select appropriate garments to wear. Children may be expected to eat healthy foods. In turn they may prepare their lunch, selecting the correct food items. The successful accomplishment of such basic daily needs engender a sense of independence and self-assurance.

Social comparison is yet another significant mechanism which influences self-image and self-esteem. As part of their interaction with their peers, children tend to compare themselves to those they meet. They observe others' physical appearance, clothing styles, modes of communication, academic performance, activities, and general behavior. These observations serve as sources of comparison. Children may gauge their strengths and weaknesses based on such evaluations. Their perceptions of their own physical appearance, academic achievement, sports performance, and social acceptance are colored by what they see and hear as they mingle with their peers. We do not like to view ourselves as losers. In order to avoid negative self-perceptions, children often resort to a variety of badly chosen *defense mechanisms*. They may decide to "give up" trying harder in certain subjects. They may refrain from engaging in sport activities. They may stop attempting to make friends. In an effort to preserve their positive self-esteem, some children gravitate toward those whom they judge to be less socially or scholastically successful. Similarly, some children may resort to outwardly belittle others, or ridicule and make fun of others' frailties and weaknesses. Hostile criticisms of others' looks, dressing habits, manner of speech or general comportment serve to elevate one's self-regard. School officials and parents need to actively prohibit this type of insulting behavior. It is the duty of both parents and teachers to enlighten children about the realities of the differences in individual personalities and abilities. We all have strengths and weaknesses. Good citizenship calls for tolerance and unconditional acceptance of others. Helping others overcome their weaknesses is an important lesson for children to learn.

Excessively shy or aggressive children may need parental guidance and supervision with regard to social behavior. Encouraging children to invite one or two friends over to their house is a good way to facilitate the learning of social skills needed to initiate and maintain friendships. Arranging for outings on weekends to parks, zoos, or museums with two or three classmates similarly promotes opportunities for socialization. Participation in sports is recommended as well. Proper sportsmanship requires civilized behavior.

SECTION 2.6:
PARENTING DURING THE YEARS OF ADOLESCENCE

The following topics are discussed in this section:
The process of individuation and identity formation
Parental support and skills needed to facilitate smooth
transition from childhood to adolescence
Risk management during the teenage years

The adolescent years span from age 13 through age 18. While responsible parenting is never an easy task, managing teenagers is an especially trying undertaking. During this phase of development individuals change in many ways. Physically children gradually begin to look like adults. Boys become more muscular, their voice deepens and facial hair begins to show. Girls become more curvacious and their breasts keep developing. These changes culminate in the achievement of sexual maturation and the capability to reproduce. As hormonal modifications take place attraction to the opposite sex becomes pronounced. The awareness of these biological changes introduces new challenges, and calls for a variety of adaptive coping mechanisms on the part of adolescents. Interest in befriending the opposite sex and experimenting with romantic overtures necessitates the learning of appropriate social behaviors on the part of boys and girls. Courtship and the acceptance of romantic advances involve sensitivities for the social and psychological needs of each other.

Awareness of responsible sexual behavior is of essence as well. On the psychosocial level teenagers become eager to assume the role of adults. At this stage of life adolescents typically find ways of defining who they are. This entails major modifications of their personalities. As they work on carving out their identities they develop a heightened awareness of their family dynamics, the social and political structure in which they function, and the religious establishments to which they belong. They evaluate their social lives, and attempt to hammer out a road to follow for a productive style of life leading to eventual financial self-sufficiency. They wish to become emancipated, and free themselves from the shackles of parental restrictions. A part-time job, which does not interfere with schoolwork, is advisable to promote gradual financial freedom. It is normal for teenagers to view themselves as grown up individuals capable of making their own decisions and pursue their activities in an independent fashion. Yet this is how conflicts arise at home. Parents feel that adolescents are in many ways inexperienced and still need guidance. They believe that the transition to adulthood needs to be gradual in order to assure safety and common sense.

In order to attain compromise between parents and teenagers it is necessary to establish ongoing open and honest communication. While adolescents need their space to experiment with the realities of life, they should heed parental advice and reasonable guidance. Finding this middle ground is a delicate matter requiring patience and understanding between daughters, sons and parents. It is wise for parents to put into practice an advisory role as adolescents vie for increasing autonomy. A dictatorial family atmosphere may create hostility and rebellion. Unless imminent danger is involved, adolescents need the freedom to test their expectations and methods of dealing with emerging challenges. It is healthy at this age to be idealistic, and to question the status quo. It is good to express political views and to debate religious dogma. It is fine to courteously question parental recommendations, values, and the "rules of the house". This is a time of transition when teenagers begin to develop their taste in music, dance, sports, clothing, and friendships.

The need for conformity to current social trends often serves as the driving force behind this period of transformation. It is at this time when intimate relationships between boys and girls may be sparked. This is the time when they express their preferences for academic or vocational subject matters. Of course these tastes and preferences may change again and again. But fathers and mothers must allow this process to take its course, and adapt their parenting styles accordingly. This entails the gradual relinquishing of control and allowing *individuation* (the formation and definition of the self) to unfold naturally, while at the same time providing love, and offering support and advice as needed to minimize potential physical or psychological mishaps. As some parents and adolescents may have difficulties adjusting to these developmental pressures, professional help from psychologists and family therapists may prove to be useful.

Undeniably adolescents are at risk for certain dangers as they depart from their years of childhood. They need to be counseled about the proper balance between their school responsibilities and their newly discovered social life. They must learn to respect essential priorities for continued academic or vocational success to meet future goals. They must be reminded about healthy eating patterns, defensive driving habits, and responsible sexual behaviors. They need to be mindful about unwanted pregnancy, sexually transmitted diseases, and the wisdom of using condoms. Dangers related to cigarette smoking, alcohol consumption, and substance abuse must be discussed. Teen-age girls frequently engage in excessive dieting to "keep in shape", and to be sexually desirable. This unsafe practice should be discouraged. There is a high prevalence of eating disorders such as anorexia nervosa and bulimia nervosa. The trials and tribulations associated with individuation and identity formation frequently give rise to clinical depression and suicidal thoughts among adolescents. Parents must be familiar with the signs and symptoms of these disorders and promptly seek professional help (See the section on mental disorders in this book).

CHAPTER THREE:

The Journey Through Adulthood

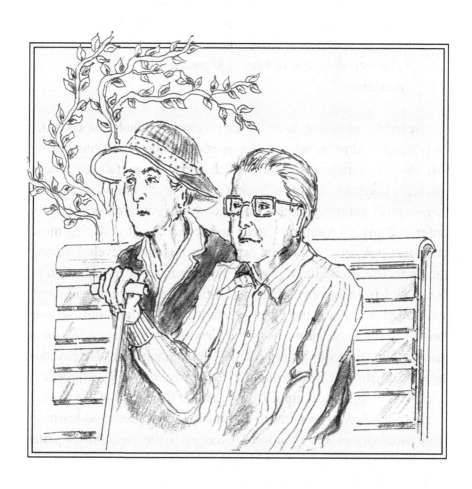

*"One of the signs of passing youth
is the birth of a sense of fellowship
with other human beings as we
take our place among them."*
VIRGINIA WOOLF

SECTION 3.1:
EARLY ADULTHOOD

The following topics are discussed in this section:
The transition from adolescence to adulthood
Career selection in early adulthood
The establishment of marriage and family life in early
adulthood

Generally speaking most developmental psychologist consider early adulthood to be between the ages of 18 and 40. Events during this span of years involve tasks, which impact many future decades or even a lifetime. Therefore insight related to the knowledge of the self, careful planning, and a realistic worldview are necessary in order to enjoy a successful career and social life. It is during these years that *independence* is first experienced on many levels. Leaving the protective umbrella of parents, completing college education or vocational training, engaging in full-time employment leading to self-sustenance mark the onset of adult life. Furthermore, serious long-term romantic intimacy with a view to establishing a family is also a hallmark of this period of life. These changes involve psychological adjustments, which ought to result in *emotional and intellectual fulfillment*. The continued enjoyment of this sense of "living life to the fullest" requires mindful monitoring of progress and learning from successes as well as failures. Changes in the execution of plans may be needed to assure continued achievement and satisfaction. The exploration of new opportunities and experimentation with new adaptive strategies may become stressful.

Excessive stress should be avoided in order to maintain optimal physical and psychological health. Maladaptive stress-reducing strategies such as drug or alcohol abuse, overeating, or cigarette smoking must be prevented. Normal hours of sleep requirements should not be reduced. A healthy diet, regular exercise, responsible sexual behavior, recreational and social activities need to be balanced with work and educational tasks. Selecting a vocation can be a difficult endeavor.

In choosing a career, personality factors need to be considered. For example, an outgoing extraverted type of person may not be suitable for a laboratory work, which entails looking into a microscope for long hours on a daily basis. Intellectual factors also need to be evaluated. For instance, a person who never attained good grades in mathematics should not seek a profession in engineering or physics. Women who expect to get married and to have several children may wish to select the type of occupation which will allow them flexible and shorter work hours. When in doubt about career selection, professional advisement should be sought. Industrial psychologists and counseling services are available for career guidance. These are listed in Appendix XX. It is a tradition in the United States to push our children toward higher education. This convention is certainly respectable, but not always suitable for everyone. Not all young adults are fit for college education. It should not be considered a shameful predicament to learn a vocation, which does not involve higher education. A skillful carpenter or electrician should not be respected any less than an attorney or a physician. Similarly, unskilled laborers are also needed in our society. In career selection the emphasis should be on what we are able to *do well*, and on what *makes us happy* in the morning when we are getting ready to face a day of work! Self-esteem is built upon individual ability, success, and pride in our accomplishments!

As young adults strive for independence, a supportive family system is crucial for the maintenance of emotional stability. Selecting a career and a life partner may be a trial-and-error event. It is important to have a protective net under us, as we walk the tight rope of independent living. As young adults face the trials and tribulations of reality and competition, financial problems and decision-making dilemmas may arise in this process of growth. The availability of parental advice and assistance provides the motivational and energizing elements in these decisive times.

In addition to the establishment of career paths, young adults' social life also needs to be shaped. Maintaining a social network of friends and acquaintances is necessary for a well-balanced life.

Trustful relationships provide much needed social support. Of equal importance is mate selection. Finding a romantic partner, marriage, and family planning are significant aspects of young adulthood. The process of match making can be a complicated multi-layered undertaking. Age, socio-economic status, ethnicity, religion, physical appearance, intelligence level, personality factors, educational plans, preferences in music, food, and many other variables need to be considered in this delicate course of action. Engaging in an ongoing relationship is an effortful responsibility. It requires time, abandoning certain activities typical of single living, and mutual understanding of each other's preferences and life goals. Both partners need to be respectful, supportive and caring. An empathetic and warm atmosphere is conducive for a happy lasting togetherness. Following marriage, probably the most important decision to be made has to do with having children. As part of this decision-making process it is advisable for newly wed couples to consult others who already have children. Such consultations can make decision-making and preparation for parenthood more realistic. Career plans may need to be delayed and financial planning may need to be restructured; the availability of family support may also need to be evaluated.

Effective communication including careful listening to emerging problems in a relationship cannot be overstated. Conflicts need to be resolved in a compromising fashion. Correcting problems in a consistent manner is reflective of the care and understanding that partners have for each other. Marital roles need to be defined and assigned in a fair manner. In today's world a single income is often insufficient to support a family. When two people are employed household and child-rearing tasks must be shared. Emotional expressiveness is also essential. Partners need to hear and see expressions of love. Spending so-called "quality time" with each other should not be forgotten. Showing interest in each other's work, aspirations and achievements further cements commitment. Married couples often tend to be engulfed so deeply in the daily hassles of life, that they end up paying little or no attention to each other. This is especially true after children are born. Raising children, taking care of a household, and earning a living are all time and energy consuming activities, which can pull married couples in all directions. Romance can easily erode if it is not nurtured consistently. It is wise to prevent such erosion at all cost. Husbands and wives need attention from each other. An eventual unhappy marriage can undermine the very fabric of family life.

Married couples frequently have different ideas about parental roles and child-rearing customs. These include, but are not limited to methods of disciplining, choice of schooling (public vs. parochial), special activities such as sports, dancing, music education, classes in religion, dressing, nutrition, selection of friends, and recreational activities. These issues require a meaningful discussion and the ironing out of discrepancies in a timely manner. The involvement of extended family members such as grandparents, aunts, uncles and cousins in children's lives also warrants dialogue. It is important for parents to be in agreement about basic parenting philosophies and practices in order to avoid future conflicts.

SECTION 3.2:
MIDDLE ADULTHOOD

The following topics are discussed in this section:
Lifestyle changes and responsibilities in middle adulthood
Issues related to retirement planning

The age bracket of 40 to 65 is considered middle adulthood. The physical effects of aging become progressively more apparent in this stage of life. Changes in hearing, vision, reproductive functioning, skin quality, bone strength, the tendency to gain weight, and general stress-resistance may occur. Susceptibility to serious illnesses (cardiovascular disease and cancer) may increase as well. Therefore, mindfulness related to prevention of health problems becomes important. Regular physical check-ups, exercise, avoidance of excessive stress, and sound nutritional habits are certainly advisable. Individuals with 'Type A' behavioral patterns need to be especially vigilant with regard to disease prevention. These people are typically highly driven, ambitious, goal oriented, intolerant of obstructions which impede their achievements, very competitive, not tolerant of others' weaknesses, and frequently pressed for time. They are frequently short-tempered, hostile, and display angry outbursts. A number of studies have concluded that anger, explosive behavior and hostility are closely related to cardiovascular disease (Berk, 2010). Psychological interventions, in particular the learning of anger management techniques are highly recommended for those with Type A behaviors.

As child-rearing responsibilities and associated financial requirements diminish many middle-age adults begin to engage in activities for which they had neither time nor money in earlier years. These functions may include pursuing hobbies, volunteering in various social or educational agencies, going to college, or learning new skills for alternate employment. The role of grandparenthood is also often a welcomed event for many adults. Involvement with grandchildren should be a *voluntary* activity. Adult children should not expect their parents to follow consistent and well-defined roles (e.g. babysitting) in their interactions with grandchildren. Taking care of aging and disabled parents may become a severe source of stress, if not handled realistically. Excessive time spent on direct care taking may have very negative effects on one's physical and mental health. This is especially true as one helps elderly parents with declining cognitive capacities, such as senile dementia. Procuring sufficient social and professional support is very much needed in such cases. Appendix XXI lists organizations that can be consulted.

Retirement planning is also a central aspect of middle adulthood. This too requires careful and insightful planning. Factors to be considered include family responsibilities such as involvement with grandchildren and aging parents, financial status, mutually agreed upon leisure activities with spouses, health status, living arrangements, and general adjustment to retired life. When in doubt, professional guidance from social workers and psychologists may be helpful in preparation for retirement. Local social service agencies may also be consulted. While retirement is a socially and culturally accepted and normal phase of life, it is certainly not a must. Many physically and psychologically healthy individuals choose to be gainfully employed and continue their careers beyond retirement age. This is especially true of people whose occupation is not physically taxing, who enjoy their line of work, and who are satisfied with their income. Many men and women need to feel useful and productive in their later years. Such inclinations are healthy and should be pursued. Forced retirement may result in a maladjusted form of living, and consequent depression.

SECTION 3.3:
LATE ADULTHOOD

The following topics are discussed in this section:
Behavior and lifestyle in late adulthood
The preservation of dignity in old age
How to provide help to elderly persons
Depression and suicide among old people
Hospice care for terminally ill individuals
Legal matters related to the termination of medical care

Compared to earlier years, Americans' life expectancy has significantly increased. This change is attributable to advances made in medical science and technology, and increased emphasis on public education related to proper nutrition, exercise, stress management, and many other factors concerning the maintenance of physical and mental health. In view of the natural age related decline of physiological and psychological functions, regular medical check-ups and adherence to physicians' and other health care professionals' recommendations are increasingly important in advanced age (beyond age 65). It is not uncommon nowadays for older adults to drive cars and to engage in a variety gainful, volunteer, and household activities. Therefore preventive monitoring and correction of sensory acuity (vision and hearing) is important.

Taking advantage of assistive technologies, such as specially designed computers, motorized wheelchairs, beds, bathroom devices and chairlifts are essential for improved adjustments to a range of disabilities. Orthopedists, physiatrists, rehabilitation physicians and psychologists, and physical therapists can recommend such equipment. Online information may be obtained at www.disability.gov For instance, cognitively intact individuals with impaired ambulation capacity can continue leading a productive style of life with the help of such assistive devices. The upholding of a healthy emotional state requires that all efforts should be made to help people function at their maximal abilities.

A word about helping behavior needs to be mentioned at this juncture. Oftentimes family members and close friends feel obligated to help elderly relatives perform certain chores, such as cooking, shopping, or banking. While offering assistance is a respectable gesture, it needs to be done in a carefully 'titrated' fashion. Familiarity with the quality and quantity of needed help is necessary in order to preserve the elderly person's *sense of independence*. Excessive or unsolicited assistance may undermine feelings of personal control. The perception of helplessness, uselessness, and dependence on others, sows the seeds of anxiety, depression, and even suicidal ideations.

The preservation of an active social, and if possible, a romantic life is equally vital for a healthy adjustment to advanced age. This is primarily important for men and women whose spouses have passed away. A number of studies have suggested that social support is a buffer against mental and emotional deterioration. While family members may be available for this purpose, exclusive reliance on sons, daughters, sisters and brothers may foster the perception of subjection and loss of control over one's life. A close relationship with grandchildren can be very gratifying. Moving to neighborhoods or residential communities where many senior citizens live can facilitate social engagement. Social workers can advise interested individuals about such living arrangements. See Appendix XXII for information leading to residential communities designed for aging persons.

Membership in social clubs, and religious and retirement organizations is advisable. Exploring programs offered by groups such as The Association for the Advancement of Retired Persons (AARP) may prove beneficial. Moving into institutions such as nursing homes should be a choice of last resort. Such drastic measures should only be taken in cases where a person is seriously debilitated and needs twenty-four hour supervision for self-care and medical needs. Whenever possible, home health care arrangements should be sought as an alternative to institutionalization. Generally speaking the quality of life in American nursing homes is very poor. Unfortunately, at times, there is evidence of abusive behavior on the part of staff. Residents are ordinarily idle, depressed, anxious and socially isolated. Their sense of individuality and self-regulation of daily existence becomes eroded.

End of life issues warrant some discussion. In general psychologically healthy adults place great value on life. Anxiety related to death is a normal process. The older one gets, the more real impending death becomes. Planning for this eventual reality is an unwelcome but necessary task. This involves legal matters, such as wills, burial or cremation arrangements and financial preparations for surviving family members and significant others.

While sudden unexpected 'natural' death is emotionally uneventful for the dying person, surviving relatives and friends may experience shock and painful grief. Mutual support within families and among friends becomes important in such instances. *Suicide rate* is highest among people who are 75 or older. Social isolation resulting from widowhood, loss of close friends, and neglectful behavior on the part of family members, chronic illnesses, restrictive disabilities, and low quality institutional care, are the principal causes of suicidal tendencies. Depression can be prevented and treated. Cognitive behavior therapy and antidepressant medication are effective in this regard. Recreational and activity therapies are also valuable. Prevention of social withdrawal, family support, involvement with grandchildren and great-grandchildren can sustain the will for continued living.

Terminal illnesses are common in old age. Sick people deserve to know the truth about their diagnosis and prognosis. It is unwise for family members to shield ailing women and men from the reality of their condition. As the time for leaving this world approaches dying people most often prefer to prepare themselves psychologically for this final departure. Attentive listening and the unintrusive presence of close relatives and friends are comforting gestures in the final phases of life.

Two important topics remain to be elucidated with respect to death and dying: hospice care, and terminating medical treatment. *Hospice care* is a philosophy of treatment for terminally ill patients. It is a comprehensive approach aimed to provide maximal comfort and the maintenance of self-respect for patients. Emphasis is placed on patients' medical, psychological and spiritual needs, and a meaning-ful, soothing interaction with their families. Pain management and emotional support is continually provided by specially trained physicians, pharmacists, counselors, social workers and nurses. Hospice care can take place at home or in inpatient settings. Families receive psychological support throughout this process, and even for months following the death of a loved one. Prolonged suffering as the consequence of terminal illnesses at home or in institutions is a sad and unwanted prospect for many. In today's advanced age of medical technology people can be kept alive for many months and years even given the failure of their vital organs. Many individuals have no desire for this possibility of artificially managed life. Hence legal steps may be taken for allowing medical professionals to terminate treatment of terminally ill patients. An *'advance medical directive'* is available for this purpose. In the United States there exist two recognized directives, namely a *'living will'* and a *'durable power of attorney for health care'*. Attorneys who specialize in this area of law need to be consulted. In essence a living will is designed for people to indicate which medical interventions they do or do not desire in case of terminal illness or any other near-death situations, such as airplane crashes, earthquakes, or car accidents. The 'durable power of attorney' is an authorization for the appointment of another person to make health-care decisions on one's behalf. This measure is appropriate for cases where a sick person is cognitively impaired, or is in a long-lasting coma. Family members or close friends are usually chosen for this function.

CHAPTER FOUR:

The Effects of Stress

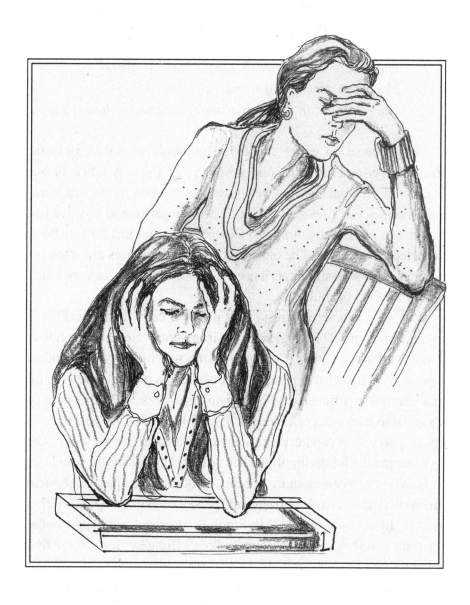

*"There is more to life than
increasing its speed."*
MOHANDAS K. GANDHI

SECTION 4.1:
INTRODUCTION, DEFINITIONS, AND BASIC CONCEPTS

The following topics are discussed in this section:
The biological, psychological, and social components of
stress
The relationship between adaptation and stress
The characteristics of stress
The relationship between arousal, motivation, and stress

Why devote an entire chapter to the topic of stress? Because stress is ever-present! It is solidly woven into the very fabric of our lives. It is unavoidable; it "welcomes" us as soon as we are born, and becomes our lifelong "partner". Both negative and positive life events can be sources of stress. Our physical and mental functions are affected by stress. The onset and course of diseases are often associated with stressful experiences. The word "stress" is very much part our daily vocabulary.

But what exactly *is* stress? Is it physical or psychological? Is it internal or external? Biological or environmental? Researchers tell us that it is all of the above. The locus of *stressors* may be found within a person (or any other organism), or outside of a person. Bodily pain, and internal experience (e.g. back pain), is a stressor. Taking care of a sick friend, an external event, is stressful as well. Our past experiences, perceptions and expectations are related to stress as well. Let us examine the following illustrative example: Mr. Smith, who lives in New York, receives an invitation, including a pre-paid round-trip airline ticket, from a close friend, to spend a weeklong vacation in his villa in the south of France. Mr. Smith is surprised and happy, but at the same time begins to feel "stressed out". But why? It turns out that several years ago Mr. Smith had a frightful experience flying. Severe air turbulence and consequent engine malfunction necessitated an emergency landing. Memories of that life-threatening incident served as a significant source of stress for Mr. Smith. His perceptions of flying, and negative expectations related to air travel were influenced by his past experiences. Mr. Smith declined the invitation.

Stress is very much related to *adaptation* to daily situational demands. Adaptation has to do with successful management of the continuous challenges we face as we go through life. Successful conquest of challenges requires effective coping skills and adequate psychological, social, and biological resources. When the necessary coping skills and resources are lacking, we experience stress. In a way we feel desperate and helpless, at least until we find suitable solutions to emergent problems.

Stressful situations often have the following characteristics: *Life transitions* involve significant passage from one life phase to another; for example, graduating from high school and starting college. *Difficult timing* relates to events which take place during time periods which are not ordinary. For example becoming pregnant, and giving birth to a child while still in school at age sixteen. *Ambiguity* has to do with indefinite or unclear events. For example, a student may be unsure of a professor's expectations regarding requirements for passing a course in college. *Low desirability* includes situations with general negative consequences or associations. For example, losing a car in a serious collision. *Low controllability* means inability to control a particular situation, such as physical or emotional pain (Paterson & Neufeld, 1987).

Stress is composed of factors which are biological, psychological, and social. Let us consider the *biological components* first. Genetic predispositions play an important role in people's susceptibility to the effects of stressors. Physiological responses to stress include increase in blood pressure, heart rate, and activation of the adrenal glands to release hormones (epinephrine, norepinephrine, cortisol) into the blood stream. At this stage the body is sufficiently mobilized to confront the stressful situation either by fighting it, or by fleeing from it. It is harmful for the body to remain in a biologically alarmed state for any length of time. Timely and effective stress resolution is therefore essential to prevent serious health problems and damage to internal organs.

Psychological factors also play an important role. Researchers in the field believe that when people are faced with stressful events, they enter into a process called *cognitive appraisal*. In other words people tend to evaluate the severity of the stressor in terms of the potential harm that it can cause to their physical or psychological integrity. This assessment process also entails a review of the resources at hand needed to tackle the stressor. Events are perceived to be *stressful* when they are unavoidable, rapidly approaching, and require a great amount of resources for counteraction. Stress often has a negative effect on cognitive processes such as attention, concentration, and memory. Sad mood, depression, anxiety, and anger may be precipitated by stressful experiences. Stress produced by catastrophic events often reduces prosocial behaviors, such as voluntarily helping others in distress. This tendency to save energy and to focus on the self may have been shaped by evolutionary mechanisms related to survival. Stress may also give rise to aggressive behaviors, such as physical fights, reckless driving, child and spousal abuse. Exposure to inescapable and prolonged stress may lead to alcohol and drug abuse.

The impact of *social and general environmental factors* in the genesis of stress is not to be underestimated. Personal relationships may be associated with stress. Incompatibility, infidelity, jealousy, psychological and physical abuse in a relationship can result in chronic stress. Family life can be equally stressful. Oppression of family members by a dominating figure, excessive control, physical or sexual abuse, alcoholism and drug abuse are causes of stress. Caring for sick or disabled family members, unemployment, and poverty are also among the causes. Divorce, single parenthood with associated financial burdens are leading causes of stress. Making a living is rarely a stress-free undertaking. Effectively dealing with the work environment often requires refined skills and even creativity. Interaction with supervisors, coworkers, and subordinates is a delicate process. Sophisticated approaches are often needed to avoid interpersonal abrasions and to mend conflicted situations. Major life events are also stressful. These include death of a loved one, immigration, moving, change of jobs, marriage, having children, facing a jail term, serious illness, and disability. Environmental disasters pose major sources of stress. Included are earthquakes, floods, fires, and nuclear accidents. In recent years acts of terrorism joined the ranks of significant stress producing agents.

As a final introductory remark we need to mention the existing relationship among arousal, motivation, and stress. We all need a certain amount of anxiety (some call it arousal or motivational energy) to gear ourselves into action. This optimal amount of arousal is highly subjective. Too little of it results in sluggishness, whereas too much of it becomes stressful. The following example illustrates this point. Some college students cannot tolerate time pressure; they find it stressful. Hence they keep up with their schoolwork throughout the semester in anticipation of the final examination. Other students need to "feel" the pressure of time in order to gain sufficient motivation to prepare for examinations. Consequently they start studying only a few days before the final examination. These students function better under elevated levels of stress. Clearly, the biological and psychological reactivity to stress, as well as the perception of stressful events are far from uniform among individuals.

STRESS, ILLNESSES, AND COPING MECHANISMS

The following topics are discussed in this section:
The relationship between stress and psychophysiological
disorders
Stress related coping mechanisms
Techniques of stress prevention

For many years in the past philosophers and scientists believed that the mind and body were distinct entities. Thanks to advances in scientific thinking we now know that the mind and the body are inseparable. They work together in good times and in bad times. A healthy body promotes psychological wellness. In the same vein a well-balanced emotional state is conducive to good physical health. When the body experiences stress, the mind is affected, and vice versa. The *diathesis-stress theory* suggests that we all have genetic predispositions to develop certain illnesses. These may be physical or mental illnesses. The actual manifestation of illnesses is very much dependent upon the amount of stress which acts upon us. For example the development of lung cancer in a genetically predisposed individual is much dependent upon the amount of stress on the lungs, such as exposure to cigarette smoke or polluted air. Stress of all sorts may increase our chances of becoming ill. Prolonged fatigue, insufficient sleep, emotional problems, unhappy or abusive relationships, personal or financial losses are just some examples.

Coronary heart disease (CHD) is caused by insufficient blood supply to the heart muscle. When the coronary arteries are blocked or severely narrowed the onset of CHD is to be expected. High levels of stress are associated with CHD. High blood pressure, enlarged heart, elevated blood clotting factors and cholesterol are all conditions related to stress. The *endocrine system* is also sensitive to stress levels. The release of the hormones catecholamines and corticosteroids into the blood stream has a negative effect on heart function and arterial blood flow. These hormones may also impair the functioning of the *immune system* (Dougall & Baum, 2001). Consequently susceptibility to disease increases. Research evidence points to relationships between psychosocial events and immune system functioning. For example, people who are more open and expressive about their problems, and receptive to available social support, often benefit from stronger immune responses. Positive emotions such as optimism boost immune functioning, while negative emotions such as depression and pessimism have the opposite effect (Kiecolt-Glaser et al., 2002).

Besides CHD there are a number of other *psychophysiological disorders* (physical illnesses associated with psychological factors). These include hypertension (high blood pressure), asthma, ulcers, irritable bowel syndrome, migraine and tension headaches, a variety of dermatological abnormalities (psoriasis, hives, eczema), and dysmenorrhea (painful menstruation) (Sarafino, 2008). Furthermore, health care providers have been expressing concern about the effect of stress on certain cancers, diabetes, and depression.

Coping with stress involves *thinking*, and *interacting* with the environment. Thinking has to do with the review of resources necessary to "deal with" the stressful event. It also has to do with the appraisal of the amount of stress at hand. Ideally there needs to be a reasonable balance between the amount of presenting stress and the required resources. Often there are a number of alternatives in managing stress. How does one decide on the "right" approach? In fact there is no uniform "right" approach! Stress management is a personal matter. It is related to factors such as personality, life style, culture, and economy. Let us consider the following example: A married graduate student with a pregnant wife is registered to take five college courses. He also holds a job as a salesman, and his salary is based on commission. He feels very stressed out because he is not getting passing grades on some of his examinations. How is he going to face this stressful situation? There are several alternatives. He can drop one or more courses and delay his academic aspirations; he can stay up late at night to study more hours and spend less time with his wife, relatives and friends; he can work less hours and earn less money. This will affect the style and quality of his and his family's life. The need for decisions of this nature are commonplace in daily life. Workable solutions depend on individual values, circumstances, priorities, and abilities.

As we cope with stress it is essential to focus on the *problem* which is at the heart of the stressor. This is called *problem-focused* coping. The above example illustrates this method. Typically when people can readily identify the problem and are confident that they have available resources to make the necessary changes, they will resort to problem-focused coping. In situations where the problems are ambiguous and people feel helpless in dealing with the stressful event, *emotion-focused* coping is used. Here people attempt to regulate their emotional reactions to stress by resorting to a variety of methods including drug or alcohol abuse, engaging in sport activities, hobbies or other distracting means such as shopping or listening to music (Berk, 2010). Some people try to summon social support in the form of advice from friends. Others prefer to view problems from a more "positive" perspective (e.g. "let this be a learning experience for me"). Still others use defense mechanisms such as denial or avoidance.

Can we strengthen our defenses against stress? What preventive steps can we take? There are a number of options and suggestions. We are all "social animals". Isolated existence is considered psychologically harmful. Social support is a powerful defense against stress. This includes family, friends, community organizations, religious affiliations, disability or illness related support groups, and professional associations. Reaching out for advice and help is a healthy process. It is a noble act to help others in trouble. It is equally important to be able to accept a helping hand when the need arises.

Another effective weapon against stress is *personal control*. Pessimism, the feelings of helplessness and hopelessness, are the "playing ground" for the devastating effects of stress. A well-developed self-esteem, resourcefulness, and an optimistic outlook on life are the ingredients for a healthy sense of personal control over life's events. Realistic *self-efficacy* is helpful when we face stress. This has to do with our knowledge of our abilities to accomplish whatever it is that we set out to do. For example, if I am out at sea in a rowboat, and a sudden storm develops, my realistic appraisal of my good rowing ability will minimize the stress related to the storm. Some practical methods are also helpful in averting stress. *Personal organization* and *time management* are examples of such methods (Sarafino, 2008). Realistic budgeting, long-term and short-term goal setting, planning for alternatives and solution oriented strategies can provide a workable framework for daily living. The use of alarm clocks, calendars, planners, tracking systems for expenses, and logical filing systems are useful items to facilitate the management of details and the organizational aspects of life. Proper nutrition, exercise, and sleep make people more resilient.

Health psychologists use a variety of techniques to help clients reduce stress reactions. Some of these include progressive muscle relaxation, systematic desensitization (counterconditioning—replacing "fear" response with "calm" response), biofeedback (electromechanically monitoring physiological responses), modeling (learning by observation), and cognitive restructuring (reducing the person's appraisal of impending harm or threat) (Sarafino, 2008). Seeking professional help is highly recommended for people who suffer from chronic stress!

CHAPTER FIVE:

Mental Illnesses

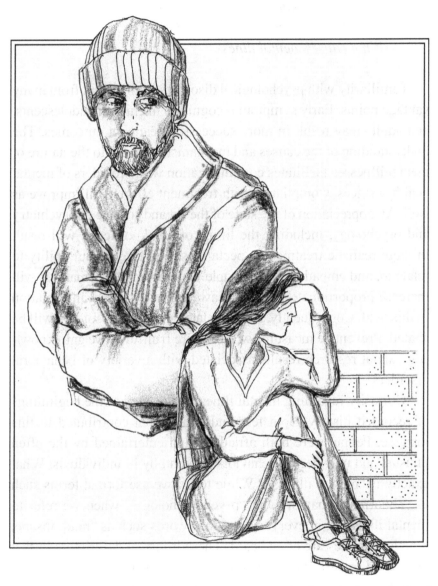

"Mental illness is nothing to be ashamed of, but stigma and bias shame us all."
BILL CLINTON

SECTION 5.1:
INTRODUCTION

The following topics are discussed in this section:
A brief historical review of psychopathology
How do we determine abnormal behavior
What causes mental illness

Familiarity with psychological disorders is important from many vantage points. Early symptom recognition in children, adolescents, and adults may result in more successful treatment outcomes. The understanding of the causes and mechanisms related to the nature of mental illnesses facilitates communication with providers of mental health services. Compliance with treatment efforts will improve as well. An appreciation of the state of the art and science of psychiatry and psychology, including the limits of our knowledge will result in more realistic treatment expectations. The level of our ability to relate to, and empathize with people with mental abnormalities will increase proportionately with our awareness of current information in this field. Consequently, stigma related to mental disorders will be abated. Preventive measures will be more fruitful as we gain knowledge about research results associated with a variety of behavioral disorders.

Curiosity regarding mental illness dates back to the beginnings of recorded history. Both fear and amusement contributed to this intrigue. People were both afraid of, and entertained by the often unusual and unexpected behaviors of mentally ill individuals. What exactly is "mental illness"? While today we use formal terms such as "abnormal behavior" and "psychopathology", when we refer to mental illnesses, in everyday parlance words such as "mad, insane, lunatic, maniac" are often heard. These informal descriptors in fact are rooted in earlier historical times. As the symptomatic manifestations of major mental illnesses have not changed over the years, both the old and modern terms describe the same types of behavioral aberrations. When talking about psychological abnormalities, the following question often needs to be answered: What do we mean by "abnormality"? Where do we draw the line between normal and abnormal behavior? While the answer to this question is not absolute, there are certain generally accepted criteria used in determining behavioral abnormality. The frame of reference in defining mental illness has not changed as we look back in the annals of history. This frame of reference has to do with the behavior, experiences and social expectations of the *average person* in a given society or culture. The survival instinct is very strong in human beings. Psychologically healthy people have a strong desire to live a comfortable long life. Hence, *self-destructive behavior* is viewed as abnormal. This includes self-inflicted bodily or mental harm, including suicidal ideations or attempts.

There are generally accepted societal beliefs and perceptions. Significant *deviations from such beliefs and perceptions* indicate abnormality. An abnormality in belief is called a *delusion*. For example if an ordinary person repeatedly insists that he is the Pope, such a belief will be sufficient to classify his behavior as abnormal. Perceptual abnormalities are called *hallucinations*. As we will later discuss, hallucinations may involve a variety of sensory modalities, such as vision, hearing, smelling, tasting, and tactual sensations. For example if a person repeatedly claims that he can clearly hear people talking to him from the moon, his claim will be viewed as a perceptual distortion, and his behavior will be considered abnormal. The communication of emotions is an important aspect of social interaction. This includes the ability to correctly identify and respond to other persons' feelings and circumstances. Unhappy events elicit the emotion of sadness; positive events elicit happiness.

Persistent inappropriate emotional reactions indicate psychological abnormality. This includes the expression of *extreme emotions*, such as fear or anger, when a more moderate level is deemed appropriate. *Repeated, sudden changes in mood* are also considered abnormal. For example, when a person characteristically expresses extreme happiness, and then changes to tearful sadness over a very brief period of time in the absence of logical reasons, such mood shifts are considered abnormal. Excessive and prolonged *emotional distress* such as severe anxiety or depression is a sign of psychopathology. *Dangerous and violent* behavior, which exceeds societal norms, is also abnormal, as are *unusual* behaviors, such as walking naked in public streets. It is important to keep in mind that *cultural factors* set the boundaries between normal and abnormal conduct. "Normal" behavior in tribal Africa, for example, is quite different from that in central Europe.

Once we understand the delineation between normality and abnormality, and the criteria used to determine pathological behavior, the next natural question to follow has to do with the explanations of mental illness. What causes mental illness? This question again has long historical roots. In primitive times unexplainable physical and mental ailments were attributed to mysterious forces entering the body. Possession by evil spirits and demonic influences were commonly believed. Madness or insanity was often considered to be divine punishment meted out as a consequence of immoral behavior. Hence, mentally ill individuals were often viewed as criminals and social outcasts. They were subjected to harsh and punitive treatment, and were housed in asylums, similar to prisons. Such beliefs and practices prevailed from ancient times through the Middle Ages, until the time of the early Greek physicians such as Hippocrates and Alcmaeon. The historical evolution of the knowledge related to mental illnesses will be further addressed in the next chapter on the treatment of mental disorders.

Contemporary scientists and clinicians view mental illness from several perspectives. It is our general understanding that human behavior is the resultant of biological, psychological and sociocultural forces. Problems arising from any one or any combination of these factors may lead to psychopathology. In the eighteenth century there were rapid advances in scientific thinking and approaches. Observation and experimentation were in the forefront as methods of research. Demonology and supernatural beliefs were on the decline. Two influential German physicians set the stage for the biological perspective of psychopathology. Wilhelm Griesinger (1817-1868) posited that diseases of the brain can result in abnormal behavior. Emil Kraepelin (1856-1926) in his famous book on psychiatry wrote that mental disorders are similar to physical illnesses in that they are both rooted in biological abnormalities (Nevid, Rathus, & Greene, 2011). Kraepelin listed mental disorders in terms of causality, nervous system involvement, symptoms, and treatment. This early classification system paved the way to the currently used *medical model*. Using this model, mental illnesses can be categorized in a way similar to physical illnesses, according to their distinctive causes and symptoms.

In the nineteenth century there were some other groundbreaking events leading to the understanding of mental illness. Some scientists claimed that not *all* forms of psychopathology could be attributed to organic etiology. It was the practice of hypnosis, which led clinicians to believe that mental illness may also be precipitated by psychological events. The famous French neurologist, Jean-Martin Charcot (1825-1893) treated hysteria using hypnotic techniques. *Hysteria* is a condition characterized by a variety of physical symptoms, such as paralysis, numbness, hearing loss or blindness, which do not have any discernible underlying biological causes. In his clinical practice Charcot demonstrated that symptoms of hysteria could be eliminated via hypnotic suggestions. He was even able to induce such symptoms in normal volunteers. The Austrian physician Joseph Breuer (1842-1925) also used hypnosis in his medical practice. It was hypothesized that blocked-up emotions, such as guilt, anxiety, or fear were transformed into physical symptoms. Talking about events associated with such emotions, when in a hypnotic state, provided at least temporary symptomatic relief (Nevid, Rathus, & Greene, 2011). Sigmund Freud (1856-1939), the founder of psychoanalysis, was very much influenced by both Charcot and Breuer. As Freud incorporated hypnosis in the treatment of some of his patients, he became aware of the importance of the *unconscious* aspects of the human psyche. The first major psychological model of abnormal behavior was based upon Freud's theory of personality development (See Appendix III). Problems arising at the various stages of psychosexual development

(Freud's theory of personality development) and the interaction of the basic components of personality (id, ego, superego) were thought to be at the core of certain mental illnesses.

The discovery of the conditioned reflex by the Russian physiologist Ivan Petrovich Pavlov (1849-1936) shed further light on the psychological explanation of mental illnesses. Pavlov demonstrated that reflexive behaviors could occur as a result of *associations*. His classical conditioning (learning) experiments with dogs proved that salivation will take place not only when food is introduced in the mouth, but also at the sight of the person who brings the food, or upon the hearing of the footsteps of the person delivering the food. It was concluded by extrapolation, that certain types of both normal and abnormal behavior could be *learned* via *classical conditioning*. Behavioral psychologist John B. Watson (1878-1958) and his associate Rosalie Rayner (1920) were able to induce fear in a young boy using classical conditioning.

Humanistic psychologists Abraham Maslow (1908-1970) and Carl Rogers (1902-1987) stated that abnormal behavior develops when people are forced to depart from their road toward personal growth or *self-actualization* (realization of our inner potentials). Having to repeatedly please others, and follow the ideas and programs of others may result in a harmful detachment from one's true self. This may lead to a distorted self-image, culminating in anxiety and depression.

Contemporary cognitive theorists Albert Ellis and Aaron Beck posited that abnormal behavior results from *irrational or distorted thinking*, such as dwelling on impending imaginary catastrophes, and generalizing, exaggerating, or obsessively magnifying the consequences of negative occurrences.

The failures of society cannot be ignored as possible contributory variables to the onset of mental illnesses. Injustice, discrimination, stigmatization, poverty, crowded and unstimulating living environments, and crime infested neighborhoods produce *stresses* which contribute to mental illness. The *sociocultural* model of mental illness indicates that social ills need to be corrected in order to prevent mental deterioration in some segments of the population.

The brain is a complicated organ, and behavior is a complicated process. Given these facts, there is certainly a lot of room for theories and views related to the causes of mental illnesses. Indeed, over the years there have been many debates in the literature as theorists were trying to establish their own points of view. As one would expect, compromises have been reached. Present day conception related to mental illness includes all three elements: biological, psychological, and sociocultural. It is called the *biopsychosocial* model. The currently used classification system of mental disorders is based upon this model. We will review this system in the next section.

THE CLASSIFICATION OF MENTAL ILLNESSES

The following topics are discussed in this section:
How we classify mental illnesses
How mental health professionals diagnose mental illnesses

Why do we need to classify mental illnesses? Scientific endeavors have to be organized to facilitate the progress of knowledge. Research and new discoveries are usually based upon the work of previous thinkers and investigators. Theories, facts and laws are categorized in a logical manner for the sake of clarification and easier communication. Classification is the core of science. The same is true for psychology and psychiatry. Patterns of abnormal behavior have to be defined and categorized in order to facilitate research and communication among clinicians.

The classification of abnormal behavior, as it was then understood, dates back to the great Greek physician, Hippocrates. Emil Kraepelin (1856-1926), the well respected nineteenth century German psychiatrist, formulated a classification system based on symptoms associated with pathological behaviors. He was the first modern theorist to propose this type of system. Kraepelin's work was very influential. In fact the system we use today is very much based upon Kraepelin's logic.

There are two manuals currently in use for the classification of mental illnesses: The *Diagnostic and Statistical Manual of Mental Disorders (DSM)*, and the *International Statistical Classification of Diseases and Related Health Problems (ICD)*. In the United States the DSM is used preferentially. The DSM was first published by the American Psychiatric Association in 1952. Since its first publication it has been revised several times in accordance with new developments in the field of mental health. The currently used DSM was published in the year 2000, and later revised. It is called the *DSM-IV-TR*. The DSM is a widely accepted classification manual in the United States of America. It is used by psychologists, psychiatrists, clinical social workers and other mental health practitioners and researchers as a guide in diagnostic formulations. It is used in private practice, clinics and hospitals, as well as by insurance companies. The DSM is not a textbook. It does not address theoretical issues related to psycho-pathology, nor does it discuss treatment approaches. It describes the course and some predisposing factors for specific mental illnesses. The focus is on symptoms, which constitute a diagnostic entity, such as "major depression", for example. The purpose of the manual is to institute uniformity and consistency in the diagnostic process. In other words, in our example the diagnosis of "major depression" may only be assigned when certain criteria have been met, as outlined in the DSM. These criteria have to do with the quality, severity and duration of symptoms, and associated functional disabilities.

As it was mentioned in the previous section, the DSM follows the biopsychosocial perspective of mental disorders. The manual recom-mends that clinicians adopt this perspective in the diagnostic process. In fact, the manual proposes a multifactorial approach, designated by five axes. Upon proper completion of these axes, the clinician can arrive at accurate diagnosis, and functional information neces-sary for meaningful treatment planning. It is advisable for informed consumers of mental health services to be aware of currently used diagnostic guidelines. See Appendix XI for a description of this multiaxial system.

In the following sections there are detailed descriptions of a selected variety of mental disorders. For a complete list of presently recognized psychiatric disorders the reader is advised to consult the current edition of the Diagnostic and Statistical Manual of Mental Disorders, published by the American Psychiatric Association.

SECTION 5.3:
DISORDERS OF INFANCY, CHILDHOOD
AND ADOLESCENCE

The following topics are discussed in this section:
The origins, symptoms and treatments of common mental
illnesses seen in infancy, childhood and adolescence
Some statistical data related to these disorders
Some preventive methods related to these disorders

In this section we will explore the major mental illnesses seen in infants, children and adolescents. We will discuss symptoms, theories and evidence related to etiology (origin and causes), and treatment approaches. In this and subsequent sections references will be made to various psychological treatments. The reader is urged to page to the chapter on psychological treatments for a full description of the various methods of verbal therapies. Similarly, references will be made to drug therapy. A full review of psychoactive medications can be found in the chapter on psychopharmacological treatment.

Before addressing specific disorders, we need to be aware of age and cultural factors as they relate to the determination of abnormal behavior. Certain behaviors may be appropriate at an earlier age, but not later in the developmental process. Some cultures and societies are more tolerant than others with regard to behavioral expectations. Stress and environmental factors need to be considered as well. Some behavioral aberrations become evident first when children begin to attend school. These behavioral changes may be temporary. The rigor of academic requirements necessitates an adjustment period. Children with no kindergarten experience may need a longer time to get used to the intellectual and social demands of school life. Boys and girls who were brought up in a sheltered fashion with little or no opportunity for interaction with children or adults other than those in their own family, may experience anxiety upon sudden separation from their parents during the first days or weeks of first grade.

Psychological disturbances in childhood and adolescence pose a serious problem in the United States. Statistics show that one in eight children suffer from serious mental disorders (Costello, Egger, & Angold, 2005). Severe depression is frequently seen in adolescents, often leading to suicidal thoughts or attempts (Pelkonen & Marttunen, 2003). See Appendix XXIII for further sources related to this topic. Risk factors for the development of mental disorders are attributable to exposure to inappropriate parenting including physical and sexual abuse, living in socially disadvantaged neighborhoods, poverty, and genetic susceptibility.

Mental retardation has two significant features: below average general intelligence (IQ of 70 or below) as measured by individually administered standardized intelligence tests, and significant limitations in adaptive functioning as measured by formal psychological assessment, clinical observation, and/or reliable and valid reports. *Adaptive functioning* refers to the ability to live independently, the ability to successfully perform self-care skills (e.g. washing, brushing teeth, dressing), and to effectively use community resources (e.g. transportation, banks, clinics, stores). Mental retardation is not an all-or-none phenomenon. There are four categories:

Mild Mental Retardation: IQ range=50 to 70

Moderate Retardation: IQ range=35 to 55

Severe Retardation: IQ range=20 to 40

Profound Retardation: IQ range=below 20

The prevalence of Mental Retardation in the United States is about 1%. Males are more frequently affected than females.

Individuals with mild mental retardation have relatively well developed communication and social skills. Their academic performance is at the sixth-grade level. They either live independently or in supervised settings, and are able hold suitable jobs later in life. Individuals with moderate retardation can benefit from training in social and vocational skills. Academically they function at the second-grade level. Under supervision they can perform unskilled or semiskilled work in their adult years. They reside in supervised settings. Persons with severe mental retardation have very poor communication, social and self-care skills. They need close supervision, and cannot function independently. Profound retardation necessitates close supervision and help with basic self-care skills, often including toileting. Usually there is severe impairment in sensorimotor functioning. Institutional living may be needed (American Psychiatric Association, 2000).

Predisposing factors for mental retardation include genetic defects, prenatal damage associated with infections or maternal alcohol consumption, perinatal problems such as oxygen deprivation, malnutrition, infections or trauma, and environmental influences such as intellectual and social understimulation, or severe emotional neglect.

Environmentally caused retardation may be reversed gradually with improved conditions, training and emotional support. Retardation of biological origin is not reversible. Special education, vocational and social skills training is recommended in most cases. Efforts should be made to facilitate maximal functioning in school, at work, and in the community. Psychotherapy may be indicated to alleviate depression and anxiety. Behavioral techniques are helpful to improve upon social relationships. In cases of severe mood or anxiety disorders, medication may be recommended.

There are three categories of *Learning Disorders*: *Reading Disorder, Mathematics Disorder,* and *Disorder of Written Expression.* Standardized tests of reading, mathematics, written expression and intelligence are used in the diagnosis of learning disorders. When a child of normal intelligence manifests significant impairment in any of these academic areas he is said to have a learning disability. Age and schooling variables need to be considered. In the United States approximately 5% of children attending public schools have been identified as having a learning disorder (American Psychiaric Association, 2000). See Appendix XXIV for additional information about learning disabilities.

Reading Disorder, also known as dyslexia, is the most common among all the learning disorders. It is estimated that about 4% of school age children in our country suffer from this disorder. The disorder is more common in boys than in girls. Characteristic features

146

include slowness in reading and errors in comprehension. Letter and word substitutions, distortions, and/or omissions are frequently seen (American Psychiatric Association, 2000).

Mathematics Disorder is seen in about 1% of school-age children. Problems may include understanding or naming mathematical concepts and operations; recognizing or reading numerical symbols; copying numbers correctly; counting objects and learning multiplication tables (American Psychiatric Association, 2000).

Disorders of Written Expression includes difficulties in any one or a combination of the following skills: composition, grammar, punctuation, spelling, handwriting (American Psychiatric Association, 2000).

Both biological and environmental influences may contribute to learning disabilities. Defects in neural brain circuitry and disadvantaged educational backgrounds have been implicated. Special education, tutoring, and supportive psychological therapies can facilitate at least partial recovery in many cases.

Developmental Coordination Disorder affects about 6% of children between the ages of five and eleven years. The disorder is not associated with a general medical condition such as cerebral palsy or any other serious neurological or pervasive developmental disorder as described below. The motor deficits significantly impair school related and essential daily activities. In younger children there may be delays in developmental milestones such as walking, crawling, sitting, or tying shoelaces. Older children may have problems with activities such as playing ball, handwriting, and assembling puzzles (American Psychiatric Association, 2000). A pediatric neurological evaluation is necessary to establish the diagnosis. Physical therapy and occupational rehabilitation are often helpful in improving coordination.

Expressive Language Disorder affects between 10% and 15% of children under three years of age. Males are more often affected than females. Prevalence rate decreases to between 3% and 7% in school-age children. By late adolescence language abilities usually show significant improvement. Proper diagnosis requires the administration of standardized instruments. Deficiencies may be manifested in both verbal and sign language. Poor expressive abilities interfere with academic achievement, occupational functioning and social interaction. Symptoms of the disorder may include any one or a combination of the following problems: limited , range of vocabulary, difficulty acquiring new words, shortened sentences, simplified grammatical structures, use of unusual word order, and slow rate of language development (American Psychiatric Association, 2000). Genetic predispositions, congenital or acquired neurological injuries, and educational deprivation may be of etiological significance. In addition to a neurological evaluation, a speech-language pathologist should be consulted for treatment options. Early intervention is usually very beneficial. Parental participation in the rehabilitation program is advisable. Parents can monitor children's progress, and reinforce proper expressive skills.

Mixed Receptive-Expressive Language Disorder has a prevalence rate of 5% in preschool children, and 3% in school-age children. Proper diagnosis requires individually administered standardized measures of both receptive and expressive language. In addition to the expressive difficulties listed above, symptoms include any one of the following problems: difficulty understanding words, phrases or sentences (American Psychiatric Association, 2000). Origins of the problems are the same as mentioned above. Early intervention as indicated above improves prognosis.

Phonological Disorder is seen in about 2% of six and seven year-olds. The disorder is characterized by a failure to use developmentally expected and age-appropriate speech sounds. Symptoms may include any one or a combination of the following problems: sound production, sound substitution, or omission of sounds. These difficulties interfere with academic and/or occupational achievement, and social interactions. Both neurological conditions and speech-motor deficits may contribute to this disorder. Early rehabilitative efforts as described above should be explored.

Stuttering is diagnosed in about 1% of prepubertal children. Boys are affected three times as frequently as girls. The disturbance is characterized by frequent repetitions or prolongations of sounds or syllables. The disturbance in fluency interferes with academic and/ or occupational achievement (American Psychiatric Association, 2000). Children with this disorder may be subjected to ridicule or social exclusion by their peers. The condition often negatively affects self-esteem. Social phobic children may further develop anticipatory anxiety related to their impaired communication style. This anxious state may in turn increase stuttering; hence a vicious cycle may develop. Professional intervention in the form of psychological counseling and speech therapy needs to be considered for accelerated improvement. Both genetic and environmental factors contribute to the development of this disorder. Social anxiety and other emotional problems may be contributory factors as well.

Pervasive Developmental Disorders are characterized by severe life-long impairments in several areas of development, such as social interaction, communication and cognition. Stereotyped behaviors and mental retardation are often present. Diagnosis can most often be made by the first year of life. Chromosomal abnormalities, structural and biochemical abnormalities of the central nervous system, as well as congenital infections are causative factors in these mental illnesses. The following disorders are included in this category: Autistic Disorder, Rett's Disorder, Childhood Disintegrative Disorder, and Asperger's Disorder (American Psychiatric Association, 2000). While a number of these disorders manifest themselves in various levels of severity, these children require special educational approaches and one-on-one rehabilitative care. Partial or full-scale institutionalization is often needed. The effects on the families involved are devastating. Professional family therapy is recommended to help parents adjust and cope with these tragedies. With few exceptions, these children will never attain independence in their adult years.

Autistic Disorder is seen in about one million individuals in the United States. Approximately four times as many boys as girls are afflicted. The onset of the disorder is before age three. The essential features of autism include impaired development in social interactions and communication and a markedly restricted repertoire of activity and interests. Non-verbal communication skills such as eye-to-eye contact, facial expressions, and body language are impaired as well. These children are often isolated socially, as a result of the above abnormalities. Language development is often delayed or absent. In those cases where language does develop, communication is repetitive, idiosyncratic, and stereotyped. There is abnormal grammar, pitch, intonation, rate and rhythm in spoken language. Comprehension is also abnormal. Children do not understand simple questions and directions. They do not recognize nonliteral aspects of speech such as humor or irony. They do not engage in symbolic or pretend play. Repetitive, stereotyped behavior is often exhibited. They have no tolerance for even minor environmental changes, such as rearrangement of furniture, variation in routine activities, clothing, or meals. Over time in some cases there may be some developmental gains, such as increased social functioning upon entering school. In milder forms of autism individuals may be able to pursue an independent style of life in adulthood despite their continued problems with social interaction and communication (American Psychiatric Association, 2000). Definitive causes of autism are not known.

A mercury compound called "thimerosal" had been used as a preservative in a number of vaccines for many years. Because mercury is a known neurotoxic agent, thimerosal was suspected to be the cause of autism by many parents. Although no scientific evidence to date has linked autism to thimerosal, since the year 2001 this compound has no longer been used in vaccines. Unfortunately the incidence of autism has not declined. Research directions focus on genetics, congenital abnormalities in neural circuitry, and prenatal exposure to toxic agents. Scientists involved in genetics research have been reporting some encouraging findings related to the etiology of about 5% of autism cases. It appears that defects on the X chromosome (one of the pair of chromosomes that determines gender) is implicated in the disorder. It is called the "Fragile X Syndrome" (Eliez et al., 2001). The syndrome is associated with abnormal synthesis of proteins related to learning and memory. As a result of this genetic failure the brain develops an excessive number of synapses (connections), many of which are immature and weak. Medications to correct this problem are currently being tested. Theoretical explanation for the mechanism of the disorder include structural and biochemical brain abnormalities, perceptual limitations, deficits in the integration of information from various senses, and hyperreactivity or insensitivity to stimulation resulting from cognitive deficits. In severe cases treatment options are limited and prognosis is poor. In mild and moderately severe cases there is more hope for partial improvement with early and intense intervention. Intensive (over forty hours per week) one-to-one behavior modification and tutoring for several years is needed to attain noticeable improvement in cognition, language, and general social behavior. In an effort to curtail aggressive behavior and tantrums, psychotropic medications are prescribed. In view of the fact that the cost of treatment is very expensive, and insurance plans rarely cover the needed interventions, many children unfortunately remain untreated.

Rett's Disorder is characterized by the development of multiple specific deficits following a period of normal functioning after birth. The disorder is only seen in females. After the fifth month of life or any time before the child's fourth birthday, changes set in. Head growth slows down, and stereotyped hand movements, such as hand-wringing begin. Interest in the social environment diminishes at least temporarily. Problems develop with muscle coordination, movement, as well as expressive and receptive language skills (American Psychiatric Association, 2000). The disorder is very debilitating and life long. As a result of the unexpected onset of this disorder the psychological effect on parents is devastating. This is especially true because at birth, and even after birth, these infants function normally. Parents are advised to seek supportive counseling and professional advice related to the type of care these children will need in years to come.

Childhood Disintegrative Disorder becomes apparent after the second year of life (always before age ten). The condition is more common in males. Symptoms include problems in any two or more of the following previously acquired areas: expressive or receptive language, social skills or adaptive behavior, bowel or bladder control, play, or motor skills. The symptoms resemble those seen in children suffering from autism. Severe impairment in social interaction and communicative skills are present. Repetitive, stereotyped patterns of behavior are evident (American Psychiatric Association, 2000). For reasons mentioned above, the psychological effects on parents is devastating. These children will require supportive care throughout life.

Asperger's Disorder is marked by sustained impairment in social interaction, and the development of restricted and repetitive patterns of behavior, interests and activities. Although language acquisition is normal, there are some deficits in communication, such as give-and–take in conversations, eye-to-eye contact, facial expressions and body language. Lack of spontaneity and initiation in social interactions is often seen. One-sided social approach to others, such as unawareness of the other person's interest in a particular topic of conversation, is a typical feature. Cognitive development, self-help skills, and general adaptive behavior are mostly normal. Males are affected significantly more frequently than females. By adolescence some individuals may learn to rely on compensatory behaviors as they become aware of their weaknesses. Consequently in their adult years these individuals enjoy gainful employment and independent living (American Psychiatric Association, 2000).

Attention-Deficit/Hyperactivity Disorder (ADHD) is probably the best known childhood abnormality in the general public. Many controversies and legal battles have surrounded this problem. There are no specific objective diagnostic psychological tests currently available for this disorder. Teachers and school administrators frequently insist on having children medicated. Oftentimes parents vehemently refuse such requirements. Approximately 3% to 7% of school-age children are affected. The disorder is more common in boys than girls. Symptoms of ADHD include any combination of the following: difficulty paying attention to details related to school work or other activities, difficulty sustaining attention, problems listening in the course of a conversation, difficulty completing tasks, difficulty organizing tasks or activities, avoiding tasks which require sustained mental effort, often losing things, easy distractibility, forgetfulness in daily activities, fidgeting with hands or feet, difficulty staying seated, excessive physical activity such as climbing or running in inappropriate settings, difficulty engaging in quiet activities, excessive talking (American Psychiatric Association, 2000). Children suffering from these symptoms may face difficulties in social situations. Their peers often do not accept them as playmates because they feel uncomfortable being around them. Conflicts often arise at home when parents insist on behaviors and limits, which these children are unable to follow. School-related problems include inferior academic performance associated with inattention and excessive disturbance in class. Teachers may exclude these children from their classes on grounds of chronic and persistent disruptive behavior. The disorder is usually first diagnosed at around age four or five. As children get older, some of the symptoms, especially those involving gross motor activity, decline in severity and frequency. Symptoms related to attention deficit may be lifelong.

Twin studies tell us that there is a significant genetic influence on the development of this disorder. Other factors include prenatal toxicity related to mothers smoking during pregnancy. Environmental factors under study include persistent family conflict, poor parenting skills, and excessive stress during the months of pregnancy. Damage to brain areas such as the prefrontal cortex (part of the cerebral cortex) which is responsible for inhibiting impulsive behavior, is being studied. Deficiencies in the neurotransmitters dopamine and norepinephrine have been associated with this condition (Nevid, Rathus, & Greene, 2011).

There are a number of medications available for the treatment of ADHD. Examples are Ritalin, Concerta and Strattera. While these drugs offer symptomatic relief, they do not cure the condition. The mechanism of action of these and other related medications are detailed in the chapter on psychopharmacology. Cognitive behavior therapy is often effective as a psychological treatment approach. When drug therapies are not combined with verbal therapies, medication discontinuation is often followed by relapse. Children need to learn cognitive coping skills to counteract tendencies for impulsive behavior. Effective parenting skills, when living with hyperactive children, involve the basic understanding of this condition. Realistic and achievable behavioral expectations need to be established. Behavior modification techniques involving immediate and consistent rewards and punishments associated with appropriate home and school behaviors need to be instituted. Close parent-teacher communication and cooperation must be maintained. Raising children suffering from attention deficit/hyperactivity disorder is difficult and may become emotionally draining. Parents are advised to attend support groups in order to share experiences, and to benefit from the successes of others in similar predicaments. Appendix XII lists information related to support groups and organizations about childhood psychiatric disorders.

Conduct Disorder involves destructive social behavior, often with serious legal consequences. Societal norms and rules are violated, including the basic rights of others. Children and adolescents who suffer from this disorder are often aggressive, and physically abusive. They may harm people or torture animals. They may steal and cause property damage. They may cheat, lie, and act deceitfully. They may set fires, run away from home, and stay out of school repeatedly. They persistently disobey authority figures such as parents and teachers. They do not benefit from punitive measures. They often belong to gangs and engage in a variety of delinquent behaviors reinforced by the culture of the gang, and the expectations of its members. They feel no remorse as their violent behaviors cause the suffering of their victims. They generally smoke, drink alcohol and use illicit drugs. Their reckless behavior frequently results in expulsion from school. Prevalence rates are higher in males than in females. Children living in urban, densely populated areas are affected more often than rural dwellers. In most cases this disorder remits by adulthood. The disorder is precipitated both by genetic and environmental determinants (American Psychiatric Association, 2000).

Unresolved parental conflicts, excessively strict parental control may be contributing factors. The modeling of aggressive behavior at home, such as violence and abusive language between parents may be associated factors as well. Disorganized family life marked by insufficient parental monitoring and communication may lead to conduct disorders. The lack of recognition and reward of children's achievements, unreasonable arbitrary harsh punishment and persistent family discord are also predisposing factors. Children who feel "lost" in the family system consequent to the lack of accountability and the absence of individual "quality time" spent with parents, may elect to join street gangs where they feel "recognized and accepted", and where their behavior, albeit antisocial, is noticed and rewarded. Their feeling of "belonging" serves as a reinforcer for continued gang membership. Treatment efforts focus on parent education.

Appropriate parenting skills with an accent on consistent rewards, punishments and well-defined accountability are taught. Positive and frequent parental interactions with their children, and the establishment of a peaceful home environment are emphasized. Some children may require anger management and conflict resolution training either in outpatient settings or in residential treatment programs. Cognitive-behavior therapy is used to enhance social skills in provocative situations.

Oppositional Defiant Disorder (ODD) is relatively common. Up to sixteen percent rate of prevalence has been recorded. A recurrent pattern of negativistic, defiant, disobedient, and hostile behavior toward authority figures is characteristic of this condition. Temper tantrums, argumentativeness, refusal to comply with the requests of authority figures, purposeful irritating and annoying behaviors toward adults, blaming others for his/her wrongdoings, excessive touchiness, resentfulness, testing of limits, and spitefulness are typical features of this disorder. Verbal aggression toward peers is also often seen. Some of these behaviors may be manifested at home, school, or any other social settings by both boys and girls. Studies suggest that this disorder is more common in families in which at least one parent has a history of mood disorder, ODD, conduct disorder, ADHD, antisocial personality disorder, or a substance use disorder (American Psychiatric Association, 2000). Sociocultural factors such as inner city stressors including poverty, overcrowding, dangerous neighborhoods, frequent crime, and availability of illicit drugs also contribute to the development of this disorder.

Children with ODD are often raised in unstable families characterized by marital discord, verbal and/or physical abuse, alcoholism and sometimes prostitution. They are often subjected to inconsistent and harsh punishments. Their parents do not provide sufficient supervision, support and emotional warmth. They are criticized often, and their achievements go unnoticed. Parental communication is poor, expectations and limits are poorly defined. Several types of treatment approaches are in current use. Social skills training, anger management and problem-solving skills have proved helpful. Cognitive therapy including modeling and role-playing with a focus on the correct interpretation of others' behavior, and thinking in terms of consequences, has been used successfully as well. Deficiencies in the neurotransmitters serotonin and norepinephrine have been implicated in aggression and poor impulse control. Psychotropic medications (antidepressants and stimulants) have been used with some success to control some symptoms of ODD.

Tourette's Disorder is characterized by motor tics and vocal tics. A *tic* is a sudden, irresistible, recurrent, rapid, nonrhythmic, stereotyped motor movement or vocalization. Examples include neck jerking, shoulder shrugging, eye blinking, facial grimacing, throat clearing, sniffing, and snorting. These expressions are unexpected, and often startling to those in the company of the person suffering from the disorder. The expression of tics results in bodily tension reduction or relief similar, for example, to a sensation experienced following sneezing. Tics are more frequent during wakeful hours. Unusual stress (e.g. excessive work load) or passive solitary activities such as listening to music may increase the frequency of tics. This disorder is usually first diagnosed in early childhood. It is believed that there is a definite genetic component to the disease, but the mode of transmission is not known at this time (American Psychiatric Association, 2000). Psychological treatments include self-monitoring, biofeedback, and relaxation training. Major tranquilizers and anxiolytic medications have been used for symptomatic suppression.

Enuresis involves repeated, mostly involuntary nocturnal voiding of urine into bed or clothes. The onset of the disorder is between five and eight years of age, with a strong genetic component (American Psychiatric Association, 2000). The disorder is more common among boys. Relaxation therapy related to frightening dreams, and conditioning techniques are used to treat the disorder. The *urine alarm* system has been especially useful: a moisture activated alarm is placed beneath the sleeping child; a sensor sounds the alarm as soon as the child wets the bed; consequently the child wakes up. Following a number of repetitions of this procedure, most children learn to wake up in response to their bladder tension prior to the sounding of the alarm. Psychotropic medications, especially antidepressants have been used with variable results.

Separation Anxiety Disorder is diagnosed when children exhibit high anxiety related to separation from parents or from those to whom the child is attached. Intense anxiety may also occur upon separation from the home where the child lives. Children with this disorder feel very uncomfortable when away from home. They often need to make repeated phone calls to ascertain the whereabouts of their parents or caretakers. They may refuse to go to school or to camp. They often fear that something tragic will happen to their attachment figures or to themselves. They fear that they will never again be reunited with their caretakers. Such fears may interfere with their ability to fall asleep. They may experience nightmares related to separation. They may insist on sleeping near their parents. Approximately 4% of children and young adolescents suffer from this disorder (American Psychiatric Association, 2000). Stressful life events, such as death or severe illness of a close relative, death of a pet, anxious parents, change of home or school environments may precipitate this disorder. Cognitive-behavior therapy, biofeedback assisted relaxation exercises, and family therapy are used to treat separation anxiety. Certain antidepressant medications in combination with psychological therapies have been used as well.

Childhood Depression is a serious and quite frequent disorder (Birmaher et al., 2006). During any given twelve month period approximately eight to nine percent of children between ages 10 and 13 experience depressive episodes. It has been estimated that about three million adolescents in the United States suffer from major depression. Girls are more at risk than boys. Symptoms of depression include self-blame for failures, hopelessness, helplessness, low self esteem, poor self-confidence and self image. Girls are often unhappy with their physical appearance; boys may view themselves as physically weak as compared to their peers. Other typical symptoms include insomnia, poor appetite, crying spells, unexplainable fatigue, social isolation, and suicidal thoughts. Children may refuse to leave the house, may be unwilling to go to school, and may show excessive dependence on their caretakers. Children may also become anxious and oppositional. Girls may develop eating disorders as a result of depression.

There are a number of explanations for the origins of childhood depression. There seems to be a relationship between children's mood disorder and parental depression. Children of depressed parents also have shown higher rates of suicide attempts than those whose parents are not depressed. These findings suggest both an environmental (learning) and a biological (genetic) component. Alcohol consumption of pregnant mothers increases the vulnerability of children to depression. Early experiences of traumatic events may lead to the development of depression in later years of childhood. Mothers as well as fathers, whose behavior is suggestive of depression, often have children who emulate behaviors such as sad facial expressions, low tone of voice, irritability, and an aloof style of interaction. Distorted mental representations, such as the persistent tendency to attribute negative events to some internal personality or intellectual defect (self-blame) are also contributory to depression. Generally speaking, children are sensitive to conflicts within the family unit. Verbal and physically abusive behavior between parents may contribute to childhood depression. Rejection by peers and insufficient parental support may elicit episodes of depression. While suicidality in children is not common, it does become a problem in later adolescence. Appendix XIII lists risk factors associated with suicide in children and adolescents. It is advised that parents should be vigilant and keep these risk factors in mind. Adolescence is a turmoil-filled phase of development.

Both social and academic stressors pose challenges for which teenagers may not have the required coping skills. Parental support and understanding is essential at this time. A friendly home environment as well as open channels of communication with teenagers is of great importance. Professional help must be procured when symptoms of depression persist. Psychological interventions with depressed and suicidal children and adolescents include individual supportive therapy, learning adaptive problem-solving techniques, stress management, cognitive restructuring, social skills training, group therapy, and family therapy. Antidepressant medications in conjunction with psychological therapies have also been used. In serious cases hospitalization may be indicated.

MOOD DISORDERS

The following topics are discussed in this section:
The meaning of mood episodes
Categories of mood disorders
Symptoms of depression and bipolar illness
Treatment modalities for mood disorders
Suicide prevention
Theories related to the causes of mood disorders

The understanding of *mood episodes* is necessary as we review the diagnostic categories of mood disorders. The *major depressive episode* is characterized by a period of at least two weeks in duration in which there is either depressed mood, or the loss of interest or pleasure in most activities. Other symptoms may include feelings of helplessness, hopelessness, worthlessness, difficulty concentrating, weight loss or weight gain, sleep disturbances, suicidal behavior (See Appendix XIV for recommendations related to suicide prevention.), low energy level, increased irritability, reduced interest in sexual activity, social isolation, low frustration tolerance, agitation, restlessness, excessive self-blame, and difficulty making decisions.

The *manic episode* is characterized by an at least one week-long period of elevated, expansive, and/or irritable mood. Additional symptoms may include decreased need for sleep, flight of ideas, grandiosity, distractibility, pressured, loud and rapid speech, inflated self-esteem, hypersexuality, excessive motor activity, increased sociability, and poor judgment in financial and social domains. A *mixed episode* involves symptoms associated with both the major depressive episode and the manic episode. The individual experiences rapid mood shifts ranging from deep depression to manic excitement. The *hypomanic episode* is defined by a period of at least four days in duration, in which there is unusually irritable, elevated, or expansive mood. Additional symptoms may be present as described above under the manic episode, but with a lesser degree of severity.

Individuals who experience hypomanic episodes ordinarily do not suffer marked impairment in social or occupational functioning. On the other hand, major depressive, manic, and mixed episodes are accompanied by significant functional impairments, frequently with the need for hospitalization (American Psychiatric Association, 2000). We are now ready to describe the categories of mood disorders:

Major Depressive Disorder (MDD): The diagnostic features of this disorder include the occurrence of one or more major depressive episodes, as described above. This is a serious and disabling disorder resulting in significant functional impairments. People with MDD are not able to complete their work or school responsibilities. They often refuse to get out of bed, feel weak, refuse to eat, and refuse to shower and get dressed. They are not interested in any social activities. They do not answer the phone, do not watch television, and talk very little. They lack motivation, and do not want to face the day. They feel hopeless and helpless, and lack the ability to enjoy life. They may be guilt-ridden, and feel that they are a burden to their families. They feel emotionally empty, and may entertain the idea of ending their life. Severe episodes of depression may include delusions and hallucinations. It is important to understand that MDD is not a sign of "weakness" or "laziness". It is a disease, which requires professional intervention. Treatment modalities include antidepressant medications, supportive and cognitive behavior therapies, and in some cases, electroconvulsive (ECT) therapy. The course of major depression is variable. It may last from several months to a year or longer. The disorder usually recurs several times during a person's lifetime. MDD is more common in women than in men. It usually develops in young adulthood. People who are separated or divorced have a higher rate of incidence than married or never-married individuals. People who are at the lower end of the socioeconomic ladder are at greater risk for developing this disorder (Nevid, Rathus, & Greene, 2011).

Seasonal Affective Disorder (SAD): This is a type of major depression (Westrin & Lam, 2007). As the name implies, this disorder is associated with seasonal changes (summer into late fall and winter). As these seasons change, some people experience fatigue, craving for carbohydrates, weight gain, and the need for excessive sleep. The symptoms fade with early signs of spring. Young adults and women are affected most. While the causes of this disorder are still unknown, there are some speculations. Changes in the body's underlying biological rhythms (e.g. sleep-wake cycles) as a result of seasonal changes in light have been implicated. Reduced availability of the mood-regulating neurotransmitter serotonin during the winter months may also be a causative factor. Exposure to bright artificial light (*phototherapy*) directed at the eyes throughout the winter season has been found to be helpful in reducing some of the symptoms of SAD.

Postpartum Depression: Following the birth of a child, some mothers (approximately 13%) experience severe mood changes, which may last for many months (Barlow & Durand, 2005). This is a form of major depression with accompanying symptoms such as sleep and appetite disturbances, difficulties with concentration, and low self-esteem. Risk factors include a history of depression, first-time motherhood, non-supportive husband and other family members, financial problems, and an unwanted or sick infant. Psychotherapy and antidepressant medications have been found helpful in treating this condition.

Dysthymic Disorder: This is a milder form of depression, but longer in duration, often lasting for years. Relapse rate is high, and slipping into major depressive episodes occurs with a very high frequency (about 90%). The disorder is more common in women than in men. Symptoms include a persistent depressed mood, low self-esteem. Impairment in occupational and social functioning is often evident. People suffering from dysthymia usually have only a very limited number of friends, if any. People find it emotionally draining to be in the company of someone suffering from this disorder. Individual and group therapies often in combination with antidepressant medications are used to treat this disorder. About 6% of the general population is affected (American Psychiatric Association, 2000).

Bipolar Disorder: This disorder is characterized by extreme mood swings from deep depression to distinct manic episodes. The first symptoms usually develop around age twenty. Men and women are equally susceptible. The disorder is very disabling, chronic, and requires professional intervention. Mood stabilizing and antidepressant medications in combination with supportive and educational psychological therapies are used to control the disorder. Support groups for family members living with the person suffering from this condition is recommended. A chronic but less severe form of bipolar disorder is known as *cyclothymic disorder.*

While the precise causes of mood disorders are not known, there exist a number of theories, which suggest some possible explanations. As is the case with many psychological disorders, *stress* is a contributory factor in the development of mood disorders. Common types of stress include loss of immediate social support, such as severe illness or death of a loved one, sudden breakup of a romantic relationship, or moving away from one's social area, as is the case with immigration. Prolonged economic hardship, unemployment, having to take care of severely ill relatives at home, marital problems, work or school pressure, legal problems and chronic physical illness and pain are also significant sources of stress. Effective coping skills, strong marital relationship, and a supportive social network such as helpful friends and relatives are important positive factors in reducing the harmful forces of stress. *Loss* is an important contributor to depression. Losing a loved one through death or separation implies loss of significant social support, which is often tied to loss of security, and self esteem. People who are "floundering aimlessly" in life may also experience depression. Such individuals lack a sense of purpose and direction. The very meaning of their existence becomes questionable. The routine and colorless nature of daily living can have a negative bearing on self-concept and self-worth, leading to despair and depression. Repeated failures in various aspects of life, such as business, school or personal relationships can also result in depression.

People, whose coping and problem-solving skills are defective, may encounter successive and perceptually unavoidable failures. These people often lack of self-knowledge of their strengths and weaknesses. They do not try new strategies to solve problems. They blame themselves for failures and develop a sense of helplessness, which paves the road to depression. Early learning experiences in childhood can lead to *cognitive distortions*, or errors in thinking such as excessive negative beliefs (inadequacies) about oneself (Beck, 1967). Chronic exposure to overly demanding parents and/or to excessively difficult academic requirements may lead to despair. Children who find themselves in such situations become hopeless. They feel that no matter how much effort they exert, they cannot "reach the top of the mountain". Hence they develop a negative view of themselves, of their environment and of their future. They typically generalize and magnify their weaknesses, and expect a life fraught with failures and catastrophic consequences. Both family and twin studies have shown that heredity plays a significant role in depressive disorders. Deficits in a variety of neurotransmitters as well as abnormalities in the structure of the brain have also been implicated in depression.

SECTION 5.5:
ANXIETY DISORDERS

The following topics are discussed in this section:
The difference between normal and pathological anxiety
Description of panic disorder
Categories of anxiety disorders
Symptoms of anxiety disorders
The difference between fears and phobias
Treatment modalities for anxiety disorders
Theories related to the causes of anxiety conditions

It is important to differentiate between adaptive (normal) states of anxiety and anxiety disorders. Normal anxiety has a motivating function, and in many cases it improves the level of our performance. Changes in our physiological state and external environmental events may cause anxiety. For example, persistent stomachaches may make us worried and anxious; hence we will be motivated to seek medical attention. When we smell smoke in the house, we become alarmed and anxious, and will be motivated to look for the cause of the problem and if needed call the fire department. A moderate amount of anticipatory anxiety will induce a student to study for an upcoming examination. When anxiety is out of proportion to a perceived danger, or when it occurs randomly in an unpredictable fashion, it then becomes emotionally distressing. Abnormal anxiety can be very debilitating, requiring professional intervention.

Panic disorder is a severe form of anxiety diagnosed in bout 10% of individuals referred for mental health consultation. Symptoms may include any combination of the following, and may last from ten minutes to several hours: accelerated heart rate or palpitations, sweating, trembling, shortness of breath, feeling of choking, chest pain, nausea, feeling lightheaded, feelings of unreality or being detached from oneself, fear of losing control, fear of dying, tingling sensations, chills or hot flushes (American Psychiatric Association, 2000). *Panic attacks* involving these symptoms are very scary experiences. People report a sense of terror, impending doom, fear of "going crazy", fear of life-threatening illness and heart attack. Frequently people experience panic attacks in crowded environments, such as shopping malls, subways, busses, or driving in heavy traffic. They develop a strong urge to immediately escape from the situation. Negative associations develop, and people actively avoid future encounters with conditions, which prompted panic attacks.

Both cognitive and biological factors are involved in panic disorders. Internal physiological sensations such as heart palpitations or dizziness of brief duration may be interpreted as an impending heart attack by panic-prone individuals. Such misperceptions initiate an automatic biological stress reaction. The release of the hormones adrenaline and noradrenaline intensifies the initial unpleasant physical sensations. The anticipatory fear of a life threatening illness in turn becomes more severe. Researchers believe that panic-prone people are unusually sensitive to minor physiological alterations in their system, which ordinarily go unnoticed by most of us. Predispositions to panic attacks have been linked to genetic factors and anxiety sensitivity. The mechanisms underlying panic disorder are still under investigation. Current theories suggest a dysfunctional alarm system in the brain, inadequate functioning of inhibitory neurotransmitters, and defective serotonin and norepinephrine (noradrenaline) receptors in the brain (Goddard et al., 2001). Cognitive behavior therapy, drug therapy and breathing retraining have been used to control panic attacks.

Generalized anxiety disorder (GAD) is characterized by excessive chronic worry and negative expectations about future activities and events, such as finances, work or school performance. Additional symptoms may include any combination of the following: restlessness, fatigue, difficulty concentrating, irritability, muscle tension, and sleep disturbances (American Psychiatric Association, 2000).

Broad generalizations about life events and consequent associations of worry across many situations can result in GAD. Unreasonable anticipation of dire consequences to trivial matters may trigger anxiety as well. Some people may have unjustified negative outlook or persistent pessimistic beliefs about a variety of activities and circumstances in life. Distorted cognitions of this sort have an arousing effect, resulting in anxiety. We often label people with these symptoms as chronic "worriers". Defective functioning of neurotransmitters involved in the regulation of emotional states may contribute to the etiology of this disorder. Combinations of behavior therapy and drug therapy have been used to control the symptoms associated with GAD.

Phobic disorders involve chronic, often lifelong, persistent and disabling fears of specific situations or objects. While *fear* is considered to be a normal (adaptive) form of anxiety related to threat, phobias are excessive fears, which are well out of proportion with perceived threats. The emotion of fear has a self-protective function. It motivates us to take action such as fighting or fleeing. Phobias on the other hand cause emotional distress, including symptoms of panic, increased heart rate, shortness of breath, and fear of losing control. Children often experience uncontrollable crying, and tantrums when faced with phobic events. Frequently feared objects and situations include animals, blood, injection, tunnels, bridges, elevators, flying, enclosed spaces, heights, and deep water. Most adults realize that their fears are excessive and unreasonable, but they feel helpless about their condition.

Agoraphobia can be unusually disabling. In severe cases people do not leave their homes for extended periods of time. Essential symptoms include fear of situations from which it is difficult or embarrassing to escape, such as house parties, offices, trains, busses, boats, or crowded stores. Crossing bridges, tunnels, or being in crowded streets may also precipitate phobic anxiety. *Social phobia* can severely restrict a person's daily functioning. Symptoms include an intense fear of social situations. Fear of public speaking, eating in public, and meeting new people are common. People suffering from social phobia are excessively concerned about being judged negatively by others (evaluation anxiety); consequently they avoid situations where others could form untoward opinions about them, or make fun of their behavior. The disorder is more common among women than men.

Several theories and some research evidence indicate that phobias develop via a variety of learning principles. Fears are learned through the process of *classical conditioning* whereby originally innocuous situations or objects can acquire the capacity of evoking intense fear. For example, a traumatic experience with a visit to a dentist can be associated (generalized) with fear of *all* dentists, *all* dental procedures, and even with the thought of a visit to the dentist's office for a simple check-up. Such fears are maintained through the process of *negative reinforcement* (operant conditioning). Specifically, avoiding dentists and dental procedures results in reduced feelings of phobic anxiety. Consequently, refusal to have anything to do with dentists will continue. At times *observational learning* is sufficient to establish a phobic reaction. Simply observing a person having a painful experience in a dentist's chair can result in extreme fear of all dental procedures. Genetic factors and hypersensitivity in certain brain structures have been studied to better understand the biology of this disorder. In the cognitive sphere, *self-defeating thoughts* such as oversensitivity to threatening cues, overprediction of danger, and irrational beliefs have been investigated by scientists. Treatment approaches include *systematic desensitization, flooding, virtual therapy, cognitive restructuring,* (see chapter on psychotherapy) and drug therapy.

Obsessive-compulsive disorder (OCD) involves symptoms which cause significant impairment and distress. *Obsessions* are uncontrollable intrusive and inappropriate thoughts, ideas, images and impulses. Common obsessions include topics related to contamination, repeated doubts, orderliness, or sexual imagery. Some people experience aggressive impulses, such as hurting a helpless child or animal. Attempts at ignoring or suppressing obsessions are usually futile. Sometimes people try to "neutralize" obsessions by engaging in compulsive acts, such as repeated hand washing to eliminate contamination (American Psyciatric Association, 2000). *Compulsions* are irresistible repetitive behaviors such as checking to see if a door has been properly locked. The purpose of such behaviors is to reduce or prevent anxiety related to particular situations. The obsessive-compulsive syndrome is "circular" in that compulsions act as a panacea for intrusive obsessional thoughts. But soon after the compulsive act is completed, the obsessive aspects of the disease recur.

Learning theorists stress that individuals with OCD tend to be excessively focused on their thoughts, unable to interrupt the constant intrusive thinking processes which they are experiencing. They also have a tendency to magnify possible, but unlikely negative events in their lives. Such cognitive misrepresentations lead to severe anxiety, which in turn lead to compulsive acts. Accomplishing the compulsive act results in the diminution of anxiety. The psychological "rewards" gained by performing the compulsive act, will result in future compulsive activities. Genetic contributions to this disorder have been studied, but the mechanism of inheritance is still poorly understood. Structural and functional brain (frontal lobe) abnormalities are also the focus of research. *Exposure with response prevention,* a form of cognitive therapy, and medication therapy have been used to treat OCD (Franklin et al., 2000).

Posttraumatic stress disorder (PTSD) is associated with exposure to life-threatening situations, or severe injuries. Threat to one's physical integrity, witnessing events which involve death or severe injuries, or learning about unexpected serious harm to family members, close friends or associates may trigger this disorder. Some of the symptoms include intense fear, horror, helplessness, recurrent and intrusive distressing recollections of the event, recurrent dreams of the event, feeling as if the traumatic event were recurring, efforts to avoid thoughts, or conversations associated with the trauma, inability to recall an important aspect of the trauma, feeling of detachment from others, restricted range of affect (e.g., inability to have loving feelings), and a sense of foreshortened future (e.g., not expecting to have a career or marriage) (American Psychiatric Association, 2000). PTSD is often experienced by individuals who have been victims of war, ethnic cleansing, concentration camps (e.g. holocaust), natural disasters (fire, flood, earthquake), rape, armed robbery, acts of terror, and vehicular accidents.

Given some of the dominating symptoms of PTSD, psychologists believe that traumatic experiences become conditioned (associated) to previously neutral stimuli. For example, a person who had been subjected to persecution and deportation to a Nazi concentration camp in Germany, may experience severe anxiety and disturbing dreams when visiting any city in Germany, or when hearing German language spoken, or upon riding in a German-built automobile. The more severe and direct the exposure to the original trauma had been, the more severe are the symptoms of PTSD. Avoiding such anxiety evoking situations result in anxiety reduction and prevention. People who have been exposed to multiple traumatic experiences, and who have poor coping skills, and lack adequate social or professional support are more vulnerable to develop PTSD. Given that many people who experience catastrophic life events do not develop PTSD, a genetic or psychological predisposition to this condition is very likely. Cognitive psychotherapeutic techniques such as stress management, relaxation exercises, and gradual exposure training have been used, often successfully, in treating this condition.

SECTION 5.6:
SUBSTANCE-RELATED DISORDERS

The following topics are discussed in this section:
Terminology, theories and concepts related to substance
abuse and addiction
Classification of abused substances
Reasons for drug abuse
Physiological and psychological effects of drugs
Description of side effects related to chronic use and
overdose
Treatment approaches for addictive disorders

Substance use is a universal practice, and is age old. Peoples in all historical periods and across cultures have used a variety of drugs and alcohol for recreational purposes. No social dictates, regulations, or laws were ever totally successful in stopping this practice. The reason for use is quite simple: drugs and alcohol are a source of pain relief and pleasure; humans look to avoid pain, and seek pleasure. Drug use is also a social "lubricant". It brings people together as a means of social engagement. In the United States substance misuse is the most common mental disorder; it is a major public health problem. People resort to drug use in good times because it is part of "having fun", and in bad times it is a vehicle to escape from problems at least temporarily. Twenty-five percent of all deaths in our country are associated with drug use. The cost of drug and alcohol related problems is estimated to be around $300 billion. This figure includes medical, rehabilitative and crime-related expenses (Hansell & Damour, 2008). Substance abuse has a devastating effect in the work force as well. Decline in work performance and absenteeism are frequently attributed to this problem. In high schools and colleges poor academic achievement and dropout rates are also influenced by the misuse of alcohol and drugs. Binge drinking and driving in an intoxicated state cause many fatalities yearly.

There are a variety of theoretical perspectives related to drug use.

Some people have undiagnosed mental illnesses such as anxiety or depression. They turn to alcohol and/or street drugs for symptomatic relief. Genetic factors certainly contribute to drug and alcohol dependence. Alcoholism, for example, tends to run in families. Learning theorists tell us that the reinforcing properties of drugs lead to continued use. Undoubtedly the sensation of pleasure and the relief from anxiety and depression have powerful reward values. Teenagers who see their parents or friends drink or use drugs may acquire these habits simply by observational learning. The expectations that people have from substance use influence their decision to indulge or to abstain. If one is convinced that consuming alcohol will be helpful in overcoming stressful situations, then one will in most likelihood resort to drinking when faced with difficulties in life. Sociocultural factors play an important role as well. Alcohol is involved in certain religious customs. Jewish holy day celebrations, for example, include a blessing for fruit (grapes); drinking wine is part of the ceremony. In certain societies (e.g. France and Italy) wine is a conventional part of meals. In Germany and Belgium beer is a favored beverage with meals. Peer pressure in adolescence certainly contributes to drug use. Church attendance on the other hand is generally associated with abstinence from addictive substances.

Before we launch on the detailed discussion of substance-related disorders, we need to become familiar with certain key terms. *Psychoactive substances* include both drugs (prescription or non-prescription) and alcohol. These chemical agents have a biological effect on the brain, resulting in behavioral changes. *Drug abuse* denotes misuse of drugs, which may result in dangerous consequences. Some people abuse more than one drug at a time. They are called multiple drug abusers, or *polyabusers*. Chronic and repeated drug use may result in a change in body chemistry. This is called *physiological dependence* or *chemical dependence*. Individuals who are physiologically dependent are advised not to abruptly stop taking drugs. Sudden elimination of drugs may result in *withdrawal reaction*, which may be dangerous. This reaction involves highly unpleasant symptoms such as nausea, vomiting, headaches, increased heart rate, elevated blood pressure, and anxiety. Withdrawal symptoms may vary, depending on the type of drug(s) used. Over time, the initial effects of an abused drug may fade. In order to achieve the same initially experienced effect, the person must take higher doses. This is called *tolerance*, and it is associated with chemical dependence. Continued drug use leads to a "powerful need state" to ingest the drug. People feel overwhelmed and helpless, and "must have" the drug when the urge calls for it. This is called *drug addiction*. Drugs are expensive. When people run out of money to buy drugs, they often resort to criminal acts, such as armed robbery, to support their habit.

Some individuals take drugs habitually as an escape from problems, or to relieve stress and anxiety. This is called *psychological dependence* which often paves the way for physiological dependence. Classes of psychoactive substances include *depressants, stimulants,* and *hallucinogens*. *Depressants* are drugs that reduce the activity of the central nervous system. *Stimulants* are drugs that increase central nervous system activity. *Hallucinogens* are drugs that alter sensory experiences, producing hallucinations (perceptual distortions).

Alcohol is the most popular depressant. It has an intoxicating effect, with severe physiological and behavioral effects. Appendix XV lists the relationship of blood alcohol levels to behavior. In general, the more a person drinks, the more intoxicated he/she becomes. There are, however, gender differences. Women are more sensitive to the effects of alcohol. They become intoxicated at lower levels than men do. This is attributable in part to their lower body weight. Furthermore, more pure alcohol reaches their bloodstream, because they have less of an enzyme that breaks down alcohol in the stomach. The psychological effects of alcohol include impairment in intellectual abilities, memory, attention, concentration, judgment, depth perception, and orientation. Social behavior is often negatively affected as well. Inebriated people frequently overstep social boundaries. They become excessively impulsive, overbearing, sexually explicit, and aggressive. Violent criminal behaviors are often associated with alcohol abuse. Impaired judgment and slower reaction time make driving in an intoxicated state very dangerous! This results in a great number of fatalities yearly.

People who suffer from *alcoholism* are physiologically dependent on alcohol. They cannot function without a certain amount of daily alcohol consumption. *Functional alcoholics* are able to hold a job and go to school. Their family life, however, often deteriorates. They usually get drunk at the end of the day, or over weekends when they do not have to attend to their usual responsibilities. Chronic alcohol abuse leads to self-destruction. People usually lose their jobs because their drinking habit eventually affects their work performance. They lose their families because their spouses become intolerant of their behavior. Similarly, they lose their friends too. Alcohol also has destructive health effects on the liver and the brain. Extensive stiffening of the blood vessels in the liver results in *cirrhosis* (scarring) *of the liver.* This is an irreversible condition, leading to death. Manifestations of brain damage include confusion, confabulation, and severe memory losses. Genetic and personality factors contribute to the development of alcoholism. Emotional instability, impulsiveness, and engagement in high-risk behaviors are often associated with alcohol abuse. Pleasure seeking and attempts to avoid responsibilities lead to alcohol abuse as well. Observational learning also contributes to the use of alcohol. Seeing the drinking habits of parents certainly affects children's and adolescents' eventual relation to alcohol.

A variety of treatment methods are available for the treatment of alcohol use disorders. The first step is for the addicted person to realize that he has a serious "problem" which needs to be addressed therapeutically. *Detoxification* (gradual weaning from alcohol) under medical supervision is the next step. Biological treatments include medications which block the desire to drink. *Disulfiram (Antabuse)* is used to condition the person to refrain from drinking. Drinking alcohol following Disulfiram ingestion results in violent vomiting. The anticipation of this unpleasant reaction is supposed to disrupt the desire to reach for the bottle. *Naltrexone* is aimed to reduce the "craving" for drinking by blocking the pleasurable effects of alcohol. Medications are also used to reduce the side effects of short-term withdrawal in the process of *detoxification* (removal of alcohol from the body). Confrontational group psychotherapy has been found useful to counteract denial and minimization of problems connected to alcoholism. Cognitive-behavioral therapy including stress management techniques and coping skills training are useful to address psychological dependence. Psychoeducation is used to teach alcoholics the physiological, psychological and social dangers associated with drinking.

Long-term *rehabilitation programs* focus on training alcoholics to live life without resorting to alcohol. Training involves encouraging people to avoid frequenting places where alcohol is served, to refrain from befriending others who drink excessively, and to solve daily problems without drinking. Individual and group counseling are used in this process. Relapse prevention is a major part of treatment. It is important to understand that alcoholism is a serious condition, and relapse prevention must be a life-long endeavor! Self-support groups, such as *Alcoholics Anonymous (AA)* are very effective in promoting long-term abstinence. In these settings recovering alcoholics have the opportunity to share their experiences related to the difficulties of continued abstinence with others who are in a similar situation. These meetings are held seven days per week throughout the year. People in need can attend as frequently as they wish. Those who have been abstinent for a while can "sponsor" newer members. Sponsoring involves helping members to resist temptation to turn to alcohol. Support groups for family members of recovering alcoholics are also available (See Appendix XXV).

Benzodiazepines such as Valium and Xanax are highly addictive sedative agents. *Barbiturates* are very addictive depressants. Examples of these drugs include phenobarbital and secobarbital. While these drugs are available on the street, they do have legitimate medical uses as pain relievers. They are also used in the treatment of hypertension and epilepsy. Barbiturates are used recreationally because they produce several hours of relaxing and euphoric effect. In high doses undesirable symptoms include poor judgment, slurred speech, irritability, and a variety of motor impairments.

When combined with alcohol, the toxic effects may lead to death. Withdrawal from these drugs must be gradual and under medical supervision.

Opioids include codeine, morphine, oxycodone, and heroin, which are naturally occurring opiates, found in the juice of the poppy plant. Synthetic opioids include Methadone, Demerol, Darvon, and Percodan. These drugs are known as *narcotics*, because they have sleep-inducing and pain–relieving properties. They are very addictive (Nevid, Rathus, & Greene, 2011). The recreational value of these drugs is very high. They produce temporary escape from reality, and intense feelings of pleasure. Medically, opioids are used to relieve pain. The most popular and frequently used opiate is heroin. It is easily obtained from street drug dealers. The method of administration is sniffing, and injection under the skin or directly into a vein. In addition to an immediate strong rush, heroin produces euphoria, and feelings of well-being for several hours. Repeated use results in addiction.

Amphetamines are stimulants. Benzedrine, Methedrine, and Dexedrine are examples of drugs belonging to this class. Amphetamines are injected into the veins, smoked, or taken in the form of a pill. They increase the action of the neurotransmitters dopamine and norepinephrine in the brain. These biochemical changes create high levels of alertness and arousal. By stimulating the pleasure centers of the brain, these drugs also produce euphoria and pleasant feelings. College students use these drugs to maintain alertness and to reduce the need for sleep during long study hours as they prepare for examinations. When used in high doses, amphetamines have serious side effects, some of which are irreversible. These include cardiovascular irregularities, restlessness, tremors, hallucinations, and brain damage. These drugs are addictive physiologically and psychologically. Abstinence needs to be gradual and medically supervised.

Cocaine is a powerful stimulant, highly addictive, and is widely used. Approximately 15% of individuals in the United States age 12 and older have a history of cocaine use (SAMHSA, 2007). In powder form cocaine can be sniffed; in a solid form (crack) it can be smoked; in a liquid form it can be injected. Coca leaves can also be brewed and drunk, a practice often found in some South American countries. The psychological effects of cocaine include pleasurable feelings resulting from activation of dopamine (a neurotransmitter) in the brain. In high doses cocaine has dangerous side effects including nausea, convulsions, stroke, accelerated heart rate, breathing irregularities, delusions, hallucinations, depression and anxiety. Overdoses may result in lethal cardiovascular effects as heart rate increases to dangerous levels. Withdrawal needs to be gradual and medically supervised.

MDMA (3,4-methylenedioxymethamphetamine), also known as *Ecstasy*, is a powerful stimulant manufactured in illegal laboratories. It is available as a "street drug". It is a very dangerous substance, capable of producing psychotic symptoms (hallucinations), depression, insomnia and anxiety. A variety of cognitive deficits (attention, learning, memory) are also associated with the use of this drug. In high doses this drug is very toxic, and may cause death.

Marijuana is considered to be a hallucinogen because in high doses it can produce perceptual alterations and hallucinations. It is derived from the cannabis plant. It is the most frequently abused illicit drug in the United States. About 40% of individuals living in the United States who are twelve years of age or older have experienced marijuana use at least once during their lifetime. (SAMHSA, 2007) Abuse and dependence on marijuana is seen more frequently in males than in females. In lower doses it produces a relaxed sensation and mild euphoria. Chronic marijuana use results in untoward side effects, including increases in blood pressure and heart rate, problems with coordination and motor performance. It also has carcinogenic effects. Many users become psychologically dependent on this drug. There is a recent trend to legalize marijuana use for medical purposes.

LSD (Lysergic acid diethylamide) is probably the one drug known most by the general public for its hallucinogenic properties. It produces perceptual distortions, derealization, and colorful visual hallucinations lasting for several hours. Side effects include elevated blood pressure and body temperature, rapid heart rate, sleeplessness and loss of appetite. Frightful sensory distortions may be accompanied by panicky feelings.

PCP (Phencyclidine) is also known as "angel dust" in the illicit drug market. Smoking this substance produces hallucinations and states of *delirium*, which is a mental state characterized by disorientation, excitability, and confusion. In high doses side effects include convulsions, aggressive and paranoid behavior, and impaired judgment. At times comatose states can ensue.

Substance abuse is a dangerous practice. Prolonged use results in medical complications and adverse psychological and social effects. Injectable drugs carry the added dangers related to infected needles. Sharing infected needles can result in HIV, hepatitis and endocarditis (heart valve infection). Detoxification, antidepressant medications, substance abuse counseling, residential rehabilitation, methadone maintenance programs, relapse prevention training, individual and group psychotherapy, and self-help groups are the treatment modalities used for addictive disorders. A more detailed explanation of these approaches can be found in the chapter on therapeutic methods.

SECTION 5.7:
PSYCHOTIC DISORDERS

The following topics are discussed in this section:
The meaning of psychosis
The description of schizophrenia
The biological causes of schizophrenia
Treatment of schizophrenia
A description of less severe psychotic disorders

The term *psychotic* refers to symptoms such as *hallucinations* (abnormal sensory experiences such as seeing nonexistent events and hearing nonexistent voices), *delusions* (fixed, unrealistic beliefs), and disorganized speech and behavior. People who suffer from psychotic disorders are partially or wholly out of touch with reality, and have very limited or no insight into their condition, which is usually chronic and very disabling. When talking about psychotic disorders, schizophrenia usually comes to mind. It is considered a tragic and very debilitating disorder.

Schizophrenia is an illness characterized by hallucinatory experiences, delusions, disconnected and illogical thought patterns, distractibility, low motivation, difficulties with goal-directed activities, and inappropriate or flat (expressionless) affect. People suffering from schizophrenia are unable to see things from someone else's perspective. These symptoms are usually severe and unrelenting, leading to bizarre and socially unacceptable behaviors. Patients frequently claim that they hear threatening voices commanding them to perform various orders. They often report seeing frightening images. Deluded patients falsely believe that they have unusual powers and influential positions. They believe that they can read the thoughts of others, and can directly communicate with angels, god, and living things on planets in outer space. The content of their verbalizations are often poorly structured, and makes no sense. Consequently these patients live on the fringes of society, needing repeated hospitalizations or long lasting institutionalized care. Their families in general cannot tolerate their disorganized behavior, and are not willing to reside with them. Approximately 1% of the United States population has been diagnosed with schizophrenia (International Schizophrenia Consortium, 2009). The first symptoms usually occur when people are in their late teens or early twenties. The severity, and treatment resistant nature of this condition has a devastating effect on both the patient and his/her family. Over a relatively short period of time the patient becomes globally non-functional. Students drop out of school, employed individuals lose their jobs, families cannot cope, and social life breaks down.

Two general symptom patterns associated with this disease have been identified. In some patients there is a predominance of hallucinations and delusions. These are called "positive symptoms". In other cases there is a preponderance of symptoms such as poverty (very little) of speech, poor goal orientation, very low motivation, and social isolation. These are called "negative symptoms". Patients with positive symptoms generally respond more favorably to antipsychotic medications. Therefore their prognosis is better as compared to patients who exhibit mostly negative symptoms. Although there are a number of theoretical perspectives on the causes of schizophrenia, most investigators believe that defective biological mechanisms play a crucial role. Genetic factors are especially important. Children whose parents suffer from this disease have a much greater risk of developing symptoms of psychosis than those with no family history of the disease. Studies with monozygotic twins further support the hereditary influence. Excessive amounts of the neurotransmitter *dopamine* in the brain have been implicated in the development of schizophrenia. Brain imaging and autopsy studies indicate structural and functional brain abnormalities and actual loss of brain tissue in schizophrenic patients.

Antipsychotic drugs such as Thorazine, Mellaril, Prolixin, and Haldol are commonly used to control the florid symptoms of schizophrenia. A more detailed discussion on the pharmacological management of psychotic disorders can be found in the chapter on psychotropic medications. Unfortunately the unpleasant side effects of these medications often result in poor compliance. These medications reduce dopamine transmission in the brain. Psychosocial rehabilitation helps patients adjust to community life. Social skills training is aimed to improve communication skills and general social interaction. Support groups for families include education about this disease for family members who are in close contact with afflicted patients (See Appendix XXIII).

Less severe forms of psychosis include conditions such as *delusional disorder*, often characterized by persistent paranoid delusions; *schizophreniform disorder*, characterized by symptoms similar to those found in schizophrenia, but with a short duration (less than six months); and *brief psychotic disorder* consisting of one or more psychotic symptoms with a duration of one month or less (American Psychiatric Association, 2000).

SECTION 5.8:
EATING DISORDERS

The following topics are discussed in this section:
The description and symptoms associated with Anorexia
Nervosa and Bulimia Nervosa
The treatment of eating disorders
Theories and research results related to the causes of eating disorders

The DSM-IV-TR describes two types of eating disorders: Anorexia Nervosa, and Bulimia Nervosa. They are both characterized by abnormal and potentially harmful eating behavior.

Anorexia Nervosa is more often found in females than males. Approximately 0.5% of the female population in the United States suffers from this disorder. Disturbances in food consumption usually begin in adolescence in the age range of fourteen to eighteen, often associated with stressful life events. Typical symptoms include persistent refusal to maintain a minimally normal body weight, intense preoccupation and fear of gaining weight, and severe perceptual disturbances related to body size and shape. There is a heightened awareness related to food products which may cause weight gain. Total food intake is dramatically reduced, and the person's diet becomes very restricted. Self-induced vomiting, inappropriate use of laxatives, and excessive exercise are also used to prevent weight gain. Despite these unusual measures, individuals still feel either globally overweight, or "fat" in certain parts of their body, such as the thighs, buttocks and abdomen. Weighing their bodies, measuring body parts, and inspecting themselves in front of mirrors several times a day becomes and obsession. Reassurance from others that they look thin and need not continue dieting, is not effective. They lack insight into the severity of their condition, and persistently deny the potential medical dangers (impaired kidney function, cardiovascular problems) associated with their continued weight loss. The psychological aspect of this disorder is tied to self-esteem. Social pressures and the media emphasis on "keeping in shape" are very influential as well. For

182

these individuals body shape and weight determine self-esteem. Weight loss and the ability to maintain an emaciated state signify healthy self-discipline. Weight gain is equated with poor self-control (American Psychiatric Association, 2000).

The treatment of anorexia nervosa may include the need for in-patient hospitalization, where appropriate eating is encouraged and self-induced vomiting is prevented. Proper food intake is closely monitored. Underlying psychological conflicts are addressed using psychodynamic therapies. Behavior therapy is used to maintain motivation for normal eating behavior. Family therapy is needed at times to uncover and resolve pathological family dynamics, which may contribute to this disorder.

Bulimia Nervosa is somewhat more common than anorexia nervosa. The prevalence among women is about 1%-3%. The disorder is much less frequent in males. The onset of this disease is in late adolescence or early adulthood. Typical symptoms include binge eating, induction of vomiting, misuse of laxatives, fasting, and excessive exercising. Binge eating involves consuming extraordinarily large portions of food in one sitting. Preferred foods usually include high-calorie sweet items, such as chocolates, cookies, cakes, and ice cream. Afflicted people are usually ashamed of their condition. They often eat, when no one else can see them, and they lie about the amounts of food they consume, as well about their induced vomiting. They frequently experience a powerless sensation with lack of control, and even an altered state of consciousness regarding food intake. Binge eating usually first begins after a period of dieting. The fear of gaining weight associated with binge eating leads to purging (self-induced vomiting). Patients suffering from bulimia often become clinically depressed and suicidal (American Psychiatric Association, 2000). Hospitalization is needed in these cases. Cognitive behavior therapy and antidepressant medications are often the treatments of choice.

The causes of eating disorders have been extensively studied. Geneticists report that these disorders often run in families. Comparative concordance studies of monozygotic and dizygotic twins also point to significant genetic involvement in bulimia and anorexia. Abnormalities in brain chemistry have also been investigated. Low levels of the appetite-regulating neurochemical serotonin has been linked to disorders of eating (de Zwaan, 2003).

The family life of individuals suffering from eating disorders is often turbulent. This is especially true with teenage girls. It has been shown that there often exists a stressful relationship between adolescent girls and their mothers. Frequently mothers communicate to their daughters that they are unattractive and need to lose weight. Mothers may be unhappy with their family circumstances, and often struggle with their own attempts to shed some pounds. Some theorists suspect that overeating signifies feelings of neglect. It therefore may be a symbolic attempt to reach out for support and comfort. Purging, on the other hand may be an expression of unhappiness with the toxic elements of family life. In general, children with eating disorders are often the products of dysfunctional families, where they have experienced loneliness, alienation, chronic conflict, and excessive parental interference with their attempts at autonomy and independence (Minuchin, Rosman, & Baker, 1978).

In Western countries, particularly in the United States, sociocultural pressures play a very important role in the development of eating disorders. Dieting among American women in many ways is a way of life, resembling an obsession. The reasons for this endless dieting are numerous. As women play an increasing role in the workforce, they have become more conscious of their appearance. They feel that society expects them to maintain an "acceptable" body weight and shape. Those who deviate from this expectation may be at a disadvantage in the job market. The media supports this expectation in advertisements and television programs. Weight loss is big business. There are always many "new" diet programs and products promising "quick results". Health club invitations and "improved" home exercise equipments are forever being offered. Fear of weight gain is a form of anxiety for women who are dissatisfied with their appearance. Strict dieting, purging, excessive exercising and abuse of laxatives serve as "anxiety reducing agents". It is sensible to seek professional help when symptoms of eating disorders arise. (See Appendix XXVI).

SECTION 5.9:
PERSONALITY DISORDERS

The following topics are discussed in this section:
The meaning of the concept of personality
Theoretical review of normal personality development
Etiology and symptoms of personality disorders
Treatment of personality disorders

It is important to understand the *meaning* of personality before launching on the topic of personality disorders. When we talk about the "personality" of and individual, we basically refer to his/her general psychological "appearance". This is somehow analogous to a person's physical appearance. *Personality* refers to those aspects of behavior, which are relatively stable over time and across situations. For example a person who is highly organized and neat at age 25, will in most likelihood be similarly organized and neat at age 40. A person who is extroverted at age 30, will continue to be extroverted at age 50 or 60. An organized person will be organized and neat at work, at home and while on vacation. An extroverted person will behave in an extroverted fashion during meetings at work, and in family and social gatherings.

Personality covers a broad range of characteristics about a person. This includes intellectual, social and emotional domains. There are both *overt* and *covert* aspects of personality. Overt aspects are observable, such as open, friendly, and free-flowing conversations in extroverted people. Covert aspects of personality are private, and cannot be seen. Thoughts and dreams are examples of this. Some aspects of personality are *unconscious*, or hidden from awareness. Some components of personality are genetically transmitted, such as temperament, others are environmentally determined, or learned from those who were influential in the person's upbringing and formative years.

In addition to the generally accepted hereditary and environmental factors related to the formation of our personalities, there are some other determinants as well. Several personality theorists believe that our distinguishing characteristics include specific *traits* such as "friendliness", "laziness", or "intelligence". *Cultural* and *social* variables also have an important bearing on personality development. These include practices such as childrearing, education, marriage, and religion. Birth order, socioeconomic level, family size and political orientation may play a role as well.

Learning theorists claim that rewards and punishments shape our behavior. We all have a natural tendency to repeat those behaviors which lead to a positive outcome, and refrain from those behaviors which result in punishing consequences. If for example industriousness and honesty are consistently rewarded (in the context of families or cultures) during our formative years, then it is very likely that we will have "learned" these attributes, and that these traits will become central to our personality constellation.

Our understanding of the human condition, free will, self-knowledge, realistic goal setting, and self-actualization (the reaching of one's full potentials), have been emphasized by *existential-humanistic* psychologists. This view of personality development focuses on the "active" involvement of the person in the shaping of his/her personality. It is the importance that we assign to our experiences and to the meaning of our existence, which determine our psychological self.

Cognitive views regard elements of information processing as important factors in personality development. The perception, association, and retention of environmental events, as well as the self-regulation (self-reward and punishment related to goal attainment) of behavior are considered significant (Hergenhahn and Olson, 2007).

Psychodynamic theories emphasize the "unconscious mechanisms" of personality formation. Psychoanalytic techniques such as free association, dream analysis, and hypnosis are considered important in attempts to uncover the contents of the unconscious and relevant childhood experiences. Freudian theorists tell us that the root causes of our normal and abnormal behavior are mostly unconscious.

Now that we have briefly reviewed the currently available theories of personality development, our understanding of the diseases of personality will be much facilitated. Personality disorders are pervasive and of long duration. Persons suffering from these disorders are unable to function adaptively in important aspects of their lives. Their behavioral abnormalities most often affect their interpersonal relationships at work, school, with their families, and in their private social encounters. These functional impairments frequently result in significant distress, and difficulties in the achievement of educational, career and social goals. People with personality disorders frequently have a very negative effect on the lives of those living with them, or those in regular contact with them. It is not unusual therefore for seriously afflicted individuals to lead a lonely and solitary style of life. I will now describe the symptoms as found in the DSM, and causal factors of the currently recognized personality disorders. Treatment modalities will be discussed toward the end of this section.

Paranoid Personality Disorder: The essential features include pervasive suspiciousness and distrust of others. The afflicted person will doubt the loyalty and trustworthiness of friends and associates. The person will be repeatedly suspicious regarding the fidelity of his/her spouse or sexual partner. Such persons are consistently "on guard", expecting to be cheated or deceived in some way. They "look for" the validation of their most often unfounded expectations. They view themselves as "faultless" and "blameless". These faulty perceptions and attitudes frequently result in interpersonal frictions. Both genetic and non-specific psychological factors such as parental neglect and abuse have been associated with the causality of this disorder.

Schizoid Personality Disorder: Persons with this disorder are socially detached, and have difficulty expressing their feelings. They are often viewed by others as cold and distant. They are introverts and loners, often choosing solitary activities. They do not seek sexual encounters, and rarely live a married life. Cognitive theorists propose that individuals with this disorder view themselves as chronic loners who do not "need" others because they can manage life rather well by themselves. They view relationships as "intrusive and problematic".

The origin of such dysfunctional belief systems, or other causative factors related to this disorder are not known.

Schizotypal Personality Disorder: This is similar to the disorder described above. The afflicted person has marked deficits in social skills and interpersonal relationships. They have unusual perceptual experiences, odd beliefs, eccentric ideas, magical thinking, paranoid ideations, inappropriate or constricted affect, and persistent social anxiety even in familiar situations. They rarely confide in others, and have no close friends. It is believed that this disorder is related to schizophrenia, or is a genetic precursor of psychotic disorders.

Histrionic Personality Disorder: Excessive emotionality, attention seeking, and self-dramatization are the characteristic features of this condition. People with this affliction need to be the center of attention. They often display sexually seductive and provocative behavior, in their attempts to charm those around them. Others often view them as self-centered, vain, and suggestible. Their self-worth is poorly defined, and they have excessive need for social contacts and external approval. While there seems to be some genetic involvement in the origin of this disorder, systematic research is scarce in this area.

Narcissistic Personality Disorder: Individuals suffering from this disorder experience an exaggerated sense of self-importance, and entitlement. They persistently need admiration, and believe that they possess "special and unique" characteristics. They may be interpersonally exploitative and arrogant, exhibiting haughty behaviors or attitudes. They are typically self-centered, and unwilling to consider perspectives other than their own in social situations. Unsuspecting people may find these behaviors odd and even initially amusing, but eventually individuals with this disorder are not readily accepted in social circles. Psychodynamic theorists suggest that parental negligence, devaluation, and lack of proper recognition of their children's strengths and achievements may lead to this disorder. These children do not develop a normal sense of self, and lack the confidence necessary for adaptive functioning in later life. Contrary views are held by social learning theorists, who claim that narcissism has its roots in parental overvaluation and overindulgence. Such parents demand very little and shower their children with praises and material rewards when such reinforcements have not been earned. These children eventually develop a false sense of entitlement, and learn that giving and achieving are not important in life. They grow up believing such unrealistic social standards (Widiger & Bornstein, 2001).

Antisocial Personality Disorder: This is a socially harmful and potentially dangerous condition! People who suffer from this disorder have a tendency to violate the rights of others without feeling any pity or remorse. They may lie, steal, cheat, get involved in fraudulent and deceitful acts, with no subsequent sense of guilt. Aggression and violence are often characteristic of their behavior. Their illegal acts sometimes result in penalties or incarceration, but they rarely benefit from punishments, and continue to engage in antisocial behaviors. Genetic factors, general emotional deficits (defective fear and distress reactions), parental rejection and neglect have been implicated in the genesis of this disorder.

Borderline Personality Disorder: The significant aspects of this disorder are characterized by rather disabling and even life-threatening symptoms. These include self-mutilating tendencies (e.g. cutting of arms), suicide plans and attempts, feelings of abandonment, extreme mood instability, repeated unstable interpersonal relationships, poorly developed self-image, impulsivity (e.g. excessive spending, reckless driving), feelings of emptiness, and unfounded intense anger. Suggestions related to causes of this disorder include traumatic childhood events (e.g. abuse, parental loss), defective neurotransmitter functions, and damaged brain areas.

Avoidant Personality Disorder: Hypersensitivity to negative evaluation by others, feelings of inadequacy, and social inhibition are typical symptoms of this disorder. Individuals suffering from this personality abnormality fear criticisms and rejection by others, hence they avoid social events such as dating or parties, and prefer occupations where only minimal contact with people are necessary. Genetics play a role in the inheritance of temperamental inhibition. When children with such acquired temperaments are subjected to emotional abuse, humiliation and rejection by unaffectionate parents, they become likely candidates to develop this disorder (Bernstein & Travaglini, 1999).

Dependent Personality Disorder: Excessive dependence on others and fear of separation are the hallmarks of this disorder. Individuals with dependent personalities have problems assuming major responsibilities, and making decisions. They need continued approval and support. They fear abandonment. They rarely initiate activities, preferring to follow the lead of others, even in minor social contexts (e.g. deciding what movie to see). They rarely voice disagreement or discontent with others, for fear of losing friends' support. Helplessness and excessive dependence may be rooted in early childhood development. Chronic parental overprotection results in feelings of incompetence and insufficient autonomy and anxiety related to self-reliance (Widiger & Bornstein, 2001).

Obsessive-Compulsive Personality Disorder: Individuals with this disorder exhibit recurrent preoccupation with perfectionism and orderliness. They are inflexible with regard to rules, and are excessively focused on the details of their environment and the perfect scheduling of daily activities. They are extremely work-oriented, avoiding free, unstructured time. Control is essential to them in all settings. Their rigid and overconscientious sense of values and ethics make them socially undesirable. Hoarding behavior is often part of this syndrome. Causative factors related to this disorder have not been well established.

Personality disorders are typically very resistant to treatment. Traditionally, psychoanalytically oriented therapies have been used in an exploratory sense, to uncover underlying, possibly unconscious pathological psychological mechanisms, which may account for these problems. In recent years cognitive and behavior therapies as well as pharmacological treatments (antidepressant, antipsychotic and mood stabilizing medications) have been tried with limited success. Eclectic (theoretically diverse) approaches are often indicated to improve chances for improvement.

SECTION 5.10:
COGNITIVE DISORDERS

The following topics are discussed in this section:
Information related to Alzheimer's Dementia
HIV-1 infection and dementia
Description of vascular dementia
Review of amnestic disorders
Description of traumatic brain injury

Cognitive disorders are most often associated with some form of brain damage. Changes in personality may also occur consequent to the damaged brain. Damage to the brain may involve a structural (brain tissue) abnormality or a biochemical defect related to transmission of neural impulses. Several adverse events may result in brain damage. These include trauma, such as a bullet wound; a disease process, such as a brain tumor or a stroke; substance abuse, such as chronic alcoholism; poisoning, such as exposure to mercury or lead. Genetic anomalies may also result in brain damage, such as mental retardation. In this section I will review some of the more common types of cognitive disorders.

Dementia of the Alzheimer's Type: The following symptoms are associated with this disorder: difficulty learning new information or to recall previously learned information, language and motor activity disturbances, problems in planning, goal setting, organizing and abstracting information. First signs of the disease usually begins at about age forty-five, or later in life. The onset of the symptoms is usually slow, with progressive cognitive deterioration (American Psychiatric Association, 2000). The afflicted individual becomes socially withdrawn and routine bound. Creativity and tolerance for new ideas and activities declines. Impaired judgment, confusion and agitation become evident. With the passage of time the person becomes disoriented to identity, time and place. Family members' names and faces may be confused or not recognized. Personal hygiene is neglected, and contact with reality loosens. In some cases the individual may become paranoid and delusional, accusing family members and aides of trying to harm him, or to have devious plots against him. At the end stages of the disease patients become bedridden in a vegetative state. Alzheimer's dementia is an organic brain disease involving structural (i.e. deformed nerve cell terminals) and biochemical (i.e. decreased levels of the neurotransmitter acetylcholine) changes in the brain. While the nature of these abnormalities have been substantially documented, the causation is not well understood at this time. Genetic factors play a significant role in the disease.

There are no currently known treatments for Alzheimer's disease. Medications which prevent acetylcholine depletion (Aricept, Cognex), and those which regulate the activity of the neurotransmitter glutamate (Namenda) have been used with limited success. Behavioral approaches have been used to control poor self-care skills, aggression, incontinence and wandering off. Cognitive failures, regressed, infantile behaviors, changes in personality, and generally insufficient behavioral inhibition make the management of these patients extremely stressful for family members and caretakers. It is advisable to resort to professional assistance for the continued care of these patients.

Human Immunodeficiency Virus (HIV-1) Infection-related dementia: The HIV virus can damage the central nervous system. This usually happens in the later phases of the disease. The initial symptoms include diminished abilities in attention and concentration, difficulties with problem-solving ability, psychomotor slowing, and mild memory impairment. The progression of the disease is marked by increased memory impairment, confusion, delusions, disorientation, behavioral regression, withdrawal, and apathy (lack of interest). The partial success in the medical management (antiretroviral therapy) of HIV disease has resulted in a reduction in the prevalence of HIV-related dementia. As newer and more effective medications are being developed, and preventive efforts are continued, there is hope for the future elimination of this condition.

Vascular dementia: The essential symptoms are very similar to those described above. Impairments in memory, language, motor activities, planning, organizing, sequencing and abstracting are the classic symptoms. The onset of one or more of these symptoms is generally abrupt. Changes in functioning is rapid and often selective and variable in severity, depending on the affected brain regions. Mood changes, especially depression may be part of the syndrome. Diagnostic features include vascular brain abnormalities, defective reflexes, and weakness in one or more extremities (arms or legs) (American Psychiatric Association, 2000). Vascular dementia is also an organic brain disease. Insufficient or lack of blood supply to one or more brain areas is at the root of this affliction. The interruption of blood supply (oxygen and nutrient deprivation) results in the destruction of neurons (nerve cells). Medical management of hypertension and vascular disease in the early stages of the disease may prevent further progression of this disorder. As is the case with all dementias, patient care is exhausting and very stressful for family members and caretakers. Professional consultation is strongly recommended.

Amnestic disorders: Patients suffering from such disorders have difficulty learning new information (anterograde amnesia), or remembering past events (retrograde amnesia). Visual and /or auditory memory may be affected, including spontaneous recall and attentional functions. Typically procedural memory (ability to learn and remember actions and skills such as riding a bicycle or unlocking a door) is frequently preserved in these patients. Changes in mood and personality may be evident in some cases. In severe cases individuals may lack insight into their impairment. They may not realize the extent of their memory deficits, and may even deny it. Others may be unmotivated, apathetic and emotionally shallow (American Psychiatric Association, 2000).

Most amnestic disorders are organic in nature. Causes include traumatic brain injury (e. g. car accidents), strokes, toxic reactions (e.g. drug abuse or industrial pollutants), oxygen deprivation, brain infections, and chronic alcoholism. In all these cases damage or destruction of brain tissue is responsible for the ensuing behavioral deficits (Butcher, Mineka, & Hooley). Following a comprehensive neuropsychological evaluation (cognitive testing), and concurrent medical management, intensive cognitive reeducation and retraining is often helpful in the rehabilitation of these patients. In many cases patients may be able to resume normal social life, schooling and gainful employment. Individual supportive psychotherapy and motivational group psychotherapy is recommended for many patients to increase self-esteem and to promote the readjustment process. See Appendix XVI for services related to cognitive disorders.

Traumatic Brain Injury (TBI): Head injuries can be causally associated with falls, automobile accidents, industrial accidents, sport injuries, bullet wounds, and physical fights. Over two million people are affected yearly in our country. In all cases it is the actual pressure or damage to brain tissue that causes the psychological impairments. Symptoms include amnesia, cognitive weaknesses, alterations in mood, and changes in personality. Immediate medical attention followed by an extensive neuropsychological evaluation are needed in order to formulate a plan of medical and cognitive rehabilitation. Motivational therapy and social skills reeducation may be part of the treatment plan.

CHAPTER SIX:

Psychological Testing

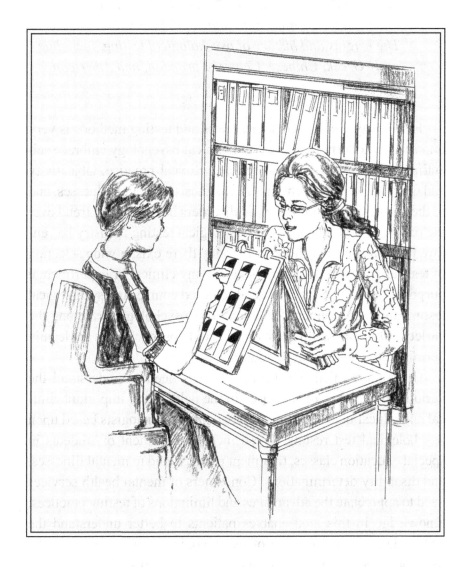

"*For most diagnoses all that is needed is an ounce of knowledge, an ounce of intelligence, and a pound of thoroughness.*"
ANONYMOUS

SECTION 6.1:
INTRODUCTION AND BRIEF HISTORY

The following topics are discussed in this section:
The need for consumers to understand mental measurement
The origins and history of psychological testing, including
early Greek, Chinese, Central European, and American
influences

Familiarity with psychological tests and testing methods is very important. Modern psychiatry and clinical psychology embrace scientific methodologies in research and clinical practice. Objectivity and quantitative approaches in the diagnosis of mental illnesses, and in the classification of psychiatric disorders have been the trend over the past several decades. The psychological testing industry has enjoyed significant growth as well. Today there exist a wide selection of tests and rating scales for just about any clinical or experimental purpose. Universities offer special required courses in psychological testing and measurement for prospective psychologists. Among the variety of mental health professionals, only psychologists are legally permitted to conduct psychological testing.

Consumers of mental health services need to understand the various applications of tests used in the field. Many important clinical and educational decisions are made by psychologists based upon psychological test results. These include placement of students in special education classes, treatment plans related to mental illnesses, and disability determinations. Consumers of mental health services need to appreciate the advantages and limitations of testing practices. Knowledge in this area enables patients to better understand the appropriateness and content of psychological reports generated by psychologists, and will allow for a more meaningful discourse about diagnostic processes between caregivers and clients.

Mental measurement has a long and rich history, dating back to biblical times. I will not attempt here to enter into the depths of this subject matter, but will briefly review some historical highlights which led to the current state of the art. The appreciation of *individual differences* among human kind is at the heart of psychological testing. Early Greek philosophers alluded to such differences in their writings. Thales (ca. 625-547 B.C.), who many believe was the first philosopher, talked about individual views and opinions about ideas, and invited others to criticize his teachings. Heraclitus (ca. 540-480 B.C.) espoused the notion that there are constant transformative physical events in the universe, and that humans are affected by these changes. Empedocles (ca. 490-430 B.C.), in his primitive theory of evolution, suggested that both animals and humans were formed randomly part by part. These random events were energized by "love" and "strife", the two essential influences of the universe. Those animals and humans whose constitution happened to be suitable and practical for continued existence survived. All others died out. The conceptualization of individual differences here is clear. Anaxagoras (ca. 500-428 B.C.) postulated that the world is a product of mixtures. Both inanimate objects and animate beings are products of this elemental mixture. Those elements in the mixture which predominate, define individual characteristics.

The prophesies of Democritus (ca. 460-370 B.C.) clearly refer to individual differences. He said that "atoms" were the building blocks of all living and non-living things in the universe. He said that the biological properties as well as the soul and mind of humans were also made up of atoms. According to Democritus, differences in biological structure and psychological function reside in the arrangements of atoms. Hippocrates (ca. 460-377 B.C.), the famous Greek founder of medicine, believed in the role of genetics and in individual predispositions to illnesses. He also talked about individual differences in biochemistry (the balance of "humors"). Protagoras (ca. 485-410 B.C.) was emphatic about individual differences in humans. He professed that it is the perception of the individual which defines truth. He furthermore emphasized that perception is influenced by previous individual experiences. Consequently perceptions can vary among the perceivers. Freedom of thought and the importance of individual opinions were central to Protagoras's convictions. Gorgias's (ca. 485-

380 B.C.) teachings were similar to those of Protagoras. He insisted that knowledge and experiences are subjective, and perceptions are private. He further posited that human consciousness is unique.

Socrates (ca. 470-399 B.C.), the famous existential philosopher, spent much time trying to explore and understand self-knowledge, the contents of the soul, and the perplexities surrounding human existence. He attached much importance to individual experiences. Plato (ca. 427-347 B.C.) was Socrates' famous student. He talked about individual variations in terms of the differential dominance of bodily needs, emotions, and reason. He introduced fundamental notions related to heredity and personality development. Aristotle (384-322 B.C.) was a devoted student of Plato. He was a very advanced global thinker, respected for his extensive contributions to knowledge in general. His insights and teachings laid the groundwork of many modern psychological theories related to motivation, sensation, cognition, memory, and dreaming. The epitome of individual differences, the process of self-actualization, was also an original Aristotlean concept (Hergenhahn, 2009).

While the early Greek thinkers created the foundations for many modern scientific developments including those in psychology, the ancient Chinese were also quite influential in paving the way for later theories related to human behavior. The appreciation for individual differences is also reflected in Chinese philosophies. In the "Book of Changes", the "I-Ching", Wen Wang (ca. 1120 B.C.) wrote about the male (yang) and female (yin) principles, ascribing activity and productivity to male characteristics, and passivity to female tendencies. Lao-tze (604-531 B.C.) discussed the virtues of those who followed harmonious living, including closeness to nature. Intellectual preoccupations were to be avoided. Confucius (551-479 B.C.) was probably the best-known Chinese philosopher. His teachings about morality served as significant markers for differences among individuals. He emphasized that honesty, trust, loyalty, and sincerity are necessary ingredients for the maintenance of prolonged family life and for successful social interactions in general (Brennan, 2003).

As we are discussing the history of psychological testing and the impact of basic Chinese philosophies on current knowledge, it is interesting to note that as early as 2200 B.C. the Chinese emperor instituted the testing of various skills in order to screen out prospective government officials who may not be suitable to fulfill such positions. These tests were designed to measure proficiencies in arithmetic, writing, music, horsemanship, and archery. Knowledge in areas such as poetry, composition, civil law, military affairs, and agriculture were also measured, using oral examinations. These civil-service tests were commonly used in China for many years (Green, 1991).

The social class system of the Middle Ages (1000-1450 A.D.) offered little room for thinking in terms of individuality. In Europe the course of people's lives were determined in large part by the social stratum in which they were born. People were molded by their predestined social environment. The expression of free will, originality, and the recognition of human uniqueness were de-emphasized until the sixteenth century. Eventually the period of the Renaissance (1450-1600 A.D.) and Enlightenment ushered in a renewed zest for knowledge. Education, scholarship, innovation, and the free exchange of ideas were again valued by society. Individualism was again respected (Aiken, 2003).

The nineteenth century was a significant period in the history of mental measurement. Scholars of that era who were interested in mental functions were typically biologists, physiologists, chemists, physicists, and physicians. They attempted to apply their traditional disciplines to the study of the mind. The earliest investigations, which ultimately led to modern scientific psychology, were in the area of "psychophysics". Of interest was the relationship between physical stimuli and subjective sensations. Ernst Heinrich Weber (1795-1878) was the first psychophysicist. He conducted his studies at the University of Leipzig in Germany, where he held the position of professor of anatomy and physiology. He became known for his seminal work on the sense of touch. He introduced methods for the measurement and quantification of sensations (Brennan, 2003). Gustav Theodor Fechner (1801-1887) was trained as a physician, but had little interest in clinical medicine. Physics became his favorite discipline. He gained recognition for his studies on sensory detection. Specifically he measured the amount of physical energy needed in a stimulus in order for it to be detectible by a person. He also investigated the changes in physical energy which was needed in order for a person to subjectively detect a change in sensation. His psychophysical experiments served as the groundwork for the understanding of the relationship between human sensations and perceptions. Another noteworthy psychophysicist was Hermann von Helmholtz (1821-1894). He is known for his work on color vision, and the physiology of the auditory system. He also studied the effect of repeated environmental experiences on the process of perception (Brennan, 2003).

German and British scientists were impressed by the work of the evolutionary biologist, Charles Darwin (1809-1882). Darwin's theory of evolution is predicated on the concept of individual differences in biological adaptability to a given environment. Influenced by Darwin's logic, scientists postulated that individual differences might reside not only in biological properties, but in psychological characteristics as well. Francis Galton (1822-1911), the cousin of Charles Darwin, was a brilliant scholar and one of the best-known British experimental psychologists. He studied the inheritance of exceptional intelligence and constructed tests for the measurement of differences in human abilities. The American psychologist, James McKeen Cattell (1860-1944) was also instrumental in the initiation of the testing movement. His research involved the measurement of reaction time in humans, and the relationship of measured intelligence with the academic performance of college students (Hergenhahn, 2009).

Interest in psychological testing was on the rise in the early part of the twentieth century. Historically significant developments took place in France. Alfred Binet (1857-1911), a self-educated researcher, became interested in the process of intellectual growth as well as many other psychological functions. As a well-respected scientist, he did most of his work at the Sorbonne. In 1903, upon reviewing the effectiveness of their educational system, the French government realized that a certain number of children were unable to benefit from mainstream teaching methods used in public schools. It became obvious that these pupils needed special education. The French government appointed Binet and his physician associate Theodore Simon (1873-1961) to assist in studying the educational needs of children with mental retardation. They created tests for the purpose of differentiating normal children from those with intellectual impairments. In conjunction with the efforts of Binet and Simon, the concepts of "mental age" and "intelligence quotient" (IQ) (as proposed by Lewis Terman in 1916) were coined by the German psychologist, William Stern (1871-1938). Henry Herbert Goddard (1866-1957) translated the Binet-Simon test from French into English. The Stanford University psychology professor, Lewis Madison Terman (1877-1956) adapted the English version of the Binet-Simon test for use with American children. Following two revisions, in 1916 the original Binet-Simon test became known in the United States as the Stanford-Binet test. Since that time, the test underwent several more revisions (Hergenhahn, 2009).

Additional developments in the testing movement of the early twentieth century include the introduction of measures of achievement, personality, and vocational interest. A more detailed review of currently used psychological tests is addressed in the following section.

SECTION 6.2:
THE SPECTRUM OF PSYCHOLOGICAL
TESTING AND MEASUREMENT

The following topics are discussed in this section:
The meaning of psychological tests
The purpose of psychological testing
Basic facts related to scientific psychological test construction
Description of intelligence tests
Description of personality tests
Description of neuropsychological tests
Description of developmental tests
Description of tests for the identification of mental illnesses
Description of psychological tests used in industry

Before the enumeration of specific tests, we need to discuss some technical matters related to measuring instruments used by psychologists. Armed with this information, consumers of psychological services will become conversant and empowered to ask pertinent questions before submitting themselves to testing procedures.

What exactly is a psychological test? Professionals define it as a "sample of behavior" which is measured in an "objective" and "standardized" manner. Let us now elaborate on these three criteria. A test is a "sample of behavior" because it only measures a specific aspect of a person's general behavioral repertoire. Furthermore, behavior is an ever-changing dynamic process. A test performance therefore is only an instance of behavior which is manifested by the testee at the time of testing. It is hoped and assumed that the "sample" of behavior is a *representative* sample from which inferences can be drawn. If such is not the case, then the test is of little value. Now let us turn to the term "objective". Scientific methods require objectivity. In the context of psychological testing this means that the scoring and interpretation of test results are devoid of subjective (personal) input by the examiner. Finally, the expression "standardized" is somewhat related to objectivity. It refers to procedural uniformity. In other words, there need to be specific documentation related to the administration of a given test, having to do with issues such as instructions given to clients, amount of time allowed for test completion, and type of materials used in the examination process. Precise guidelines related to the scoring and interpretation of tests must also be provided.

What are the uses of psychological tests? In most cases tests are used to complement clinical impressions and data gathered from subjective experiences. Examples include diagnosis of mental disorders, in clinics or hospitals; determination of learning disabilities in educational settings; and classification and placement of prospective employees in industry.

In order for a test to be of scientific and clinical value, it must possess sound *psychometric properties*. These include standardization, reliability, and validity. In addition to the definition given above, the word *"standardization"* has another meaning as well. It has to do with the establishment of *"norms"*. Norms allow us to compare the test performance of an individual to that of a *representative sample* in a specific *population*. For example, if we wish to establish meaningfully the ranking of an American born twenty-year-old person's level of intelligence, we need to know the intelligence levels of typical twenty-year-old Americans. In order for such comparisons to be possible, the intelligence test must be standardized on a representative sample of twenty-year-old Americans. *"Reliability"* has to do with consistency. Let us take a thermometer as an example. If we were to measure a healthy person's body temperature at rest, and at a certain time under specific environmental conditions, and then repeat the measurement under the same conditions, we should be able to get the same or very similar readings in both instances. As long as we are measuring relatively stable characteristics, such as intelligence for example, psychological tests must yield reliable results. Customarily *"validity"* refers to appropriateness. Does the test measure what it purports to measure? Is the test suitable for a certain purpose or situation? Is it the correct instrument for the use with particular clients? Answers to these questions give us crucial information about the validity of tests.

There are very many tests used by professional psychologists. It is outside of the scope of the present volume to review all of these instruments. The major categories of tests with examples of each are described herein. These classes include tests which measure intelligence, personality, brain damage including learning disabilities, development, psychopathology, vocational interests, aptitudes, and attitudes.

The construct of "intelligence" is known to most of us. We use the term in everyday parlance. Behavioral scientists formulated a variety of theories and definitions of intelligence. Reasoning, understanding, and judgment are often associated with the concept of intelligence. Adaptability to changing environmental demands, the ability to learn, solve problems, and to think in an abstract fashion are also significant contributors to intellectual functioning. Tests of cognitive development aim to measure these attributes either implicitly or explicitly. The meaning of the intelligence quotient or IQ is illustrated by the following formula: IQ=100(MA/CA) (MA=mental age; CA=chronological age). The concept of mental age refers to an individual's mental maturity. An eight-year-old child, for example, is expected to solve correctly those items on an IQ test, which are ordinarily correctly solved by normal (according to standardization norms) eight-year-old children. If such is the case, the child's IQ will equal 100, which is considered "average". If the eight-year-old child can also solve problems designed for nine year olds, than his IQ will be above average. Conversely, if this child cannot solve test items beyond those intended for seven year olds, his IQ will be interpreted as below average. The two most common tests of intelligence in use today are the Stanford-Binet and the Wechsler Intelligence Scales (WAIS and WISC).

"Personality" is another commonly used expression. In our daily lives we often describe others in terms of their individual attributes. For example, we may characterize people as "smart", "humorous", "friendly", "outgoing", "adventuresome", or "shy". The variety of such descriptions may indeed be inexhaustible. Psychologists conceptualize "personality" as generally consistent and stable patterns of behavior. Certain aspects of an individual's personality can only be expressed in social contexts. For example, a "friendly" person can only express his "friendliness" when in the company of others. On the other hand an introverted "home body" can easily be identified as such by observing his/her consistent solitary behavior. Our physical characteristics have many dimensions. Examples of these are height, weight, body shape, hair color, skin color, eye color, and facial features. Analogously, our personality is the reflection of our psychological profile. It includes a wide range of behavioral qualities. Many of these features are transparent and readily detectible in the course of conversations or overt actions. Others are hidden in the form of dreams, memories and private thoughts. Furthermore, the contents of some aspects of our psyche are not readily accessible because they are unconscious. Personality tests are designed to measure one or more of these dimensions. Most tests are based upon theories that aim to explain psychological constructs. Personality tests are also based on theories.

Single-Construct Inventories typically focus on one personality or symptom variable. The *Beck Anxiety Inventory* and the *Beck Depression Inventory* are examples. These are short written tests containing questions related to anxiety and depression respectively. Inventories are also used to diagnose specific mental disorders such as phobias, eating disorders, and substance abuse. Other tests measure personality traits. The *Sixteen Personality Factor Questionnaire* is an example of these. It measures traits such as emotional stability, enthusiasm, trust, imaginativeness, and self-assuredness. Probably the most widely used written personality test is the *Minnesota Multiphasic Personality Inventory (MMPI)*. The original test was designed in the early 1940's. It was revised in the 1980's. The revised version is called the *MMPI-2*. It is a so-called "criterion-keyed" personality inventory. This means that the various test items are aimed to differentiate between two or more criterion groups. This test is mostly used to identify individuals with mental disorders on a variety of dimensions such as hypochondria (excessive and abnormal concern with diseases and bodily functions), paranoia, psychopathy (serious and repeated disregard for social customs, unwillingness or inability to learn from punishing experiences), and schizophrenia (experiencing delusions, hallucinations, and exhibiting bizarre and withdrawn behavior) (Aiken, 2003).

In earlier years *projective testing techniques* were commonly used by psychologists and psychiatrists. As a result of inherent problems related to the establishment of reliability and validity, and the proliferation of behavioral psychologists, over the years, the use of these tests became less frequent. Nevertheless, projective approaches do have clinical utility. Traditionally, psychoanalytically trained professionals espouse these methods. When used by well-trained clinicians, these tests can provide invaluable psychodynamic information about patients. Unconscious motivations, needs, perceptual idiosyncrasies, feelings, and conflicts of significant diagnostic value often surface in the process of testing. Originally, patients were expected to project their inner thoughts, feelings, reactions, viewpoints, interpretations, and wishes onto undefined, amorphous stimuli presented mostly in the form of inkblots. Eventually, other varieties of projective tests were created. Construction of ideas (stories), ordering of stimuli (a set of pictures), completion of ideas (story segments), and expressive techniques (drawings) are used today to complement the associative inkblot procedures (Domino & Domino, 2006). The unstructured and open-ended nature of these tests allow for free and uninhibited responses.

Probably the best-known projective test is the *Rorschach Inkblot Technique*. It was first published in 1921 by Hermann Rorschach, a Swiss psychiatrist. The test consists of ten cards; some are black-and-white, others are colored. The respondents view the cards one at a time, and verbally report their reactions and interpretations of the inkblots. An example of the use of the construction technique is seen in the *Thematic Apperception Test (TAT)*. Here the patients/clients are instructed to relate complete stories about a variety of pictures presented to them. The stimulus cards illustrate people in a number of ambiguous situations. The test-subjects are asked to elaborate on their interpretations of each situation, including hypothetical causes and outcomes of events, and speculations about feelings of people depicted in the pictures. The *Rotter Incomplete Sentences Blank* requires the completion of sentences, which may lead to a better understanding of a person's fears, desires, needs, wishes, and attitudes. An example is: "My greatest fear is _____." Expressive techniques involve projective drawings. The *Draw-a-Person Test* and the *House-Tree-Person Technique* are examples of these projective techniques. Clients are asked to draw pictures of either sexes, several objects, or a group of people (Aiken, 2003). They may also be asked to draw a story about a house, and those who live in it. Ordering techniques require the subject to place stimulus cards, describing a story, in a meaningful sequence.

Neuropsychological tests are used to detect and measure the effects of brain damage on general psychological functioning, including learning disabilities. Common causes of brain damage include birth related complications, infections, strokes, chronic drug or alcohol abuse, trauma, genetic errors, neurodegenerative diseases, and the aging process. Consequent psychological impairments may consist of alterations in personality, and cognitive deficits involving memory, reaction time, language, calculation, attention, perceptual-motor integration, abstraction, learning, and orientation. Theoretically, any cognitive function or combination of functions may be affected. Neuropsychological tests have been designed to identify the type and extent of such alterations and deficits. The *Halstead-Reitan Neuropsychological Battery* and the *Luria-Nebraska Neuropsychological Battery* serve as examples (Golden, Purisch, & Hammeke, 1985; Reitan & Wolfson, 1993). Cognitive rehabilitation and special education plans are based upon the strengths and weaknesses of patients as indicated on the results of neuropsychological diagnostic testing.

Tests have been constructed to measure cognitive, motor, perceptual, emotional, and social development in children. Performance on these tests are indicative of psychological and motor functioning at various stages of development, also known as "developmental milestones". Early rehabilitative intervention plans are frequently guided by the results attained on these instruments. Examples of these tests are the *Brazelton Neonatal Behavioral Assessment Scale*, and the *Bayley Scales of Infant Development* (Bayley, 1969; Brazelton, 1973).

The process of diagnosis of mental illnesses must start with a thorough *clinical interview*. Typically this includes a review of presenting symptoms, functional assessment related to education, work, family and social life, past psychiatric and medical history, identification of stressors, and family history of physical and mental illnesses . This "subjective" approach is frequently complemented by "objective" diagnostic psychological tests. The aim of these tests is to detect and measure the severity of a variety of symptoms suggestive of psychopathology, such as those characteristic of schizophrenia, mood disorders, anxiety disorders, eating disorders, and personality disorders. Examples of these tests are the *Symptom Checklist 90 (SCL-90)*, the *Minnesota Multiphasic Personality Inventory (MMPI)*, the *Beck Depression Inventory (BDI)*, and the *Eating Disorder Inventory*. Repeated administration of these and other tests help clinicians monitor the course of disorders, and the efficacy of treatment efforts.

The work of counselors and industrial psychologists also involve psychological testing. Guidance in career planning involves tests which measure aptitudes, and vocational interests. The process of employee selection in industrial settings involves tests designed to predict successful performance of job applicants for specific positions. The *Strong Interest Inventory* and the *General Aptitude Test Battery* are examples of these instruments (Domino & Domino, 2006).

Finally, social psychologists and consumer psychologists often use tests to measure views and attitudes (predispositions) of people toward concepts such as political systems, educational systems, health care systems, and other services and products.

Appendix XVII lists tests commonly used in clinical practice.

CHAPTER SEVEN:

The Treatment of Psychological Disorders

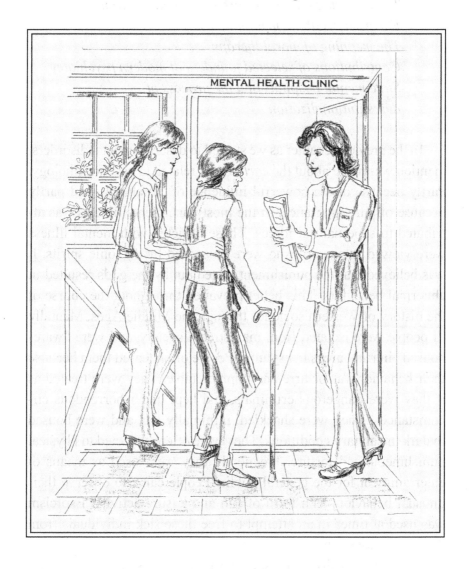

*"Natural forces within us are the
true healers of disease."*
HIPPOCRATES

SECTION 7.1:
BRIEF HISTORY

The following topics are discussed in this section:
Early beliefs about mental illness
The meaning of moral therapy
Contributions of selected founders of modern psychiatry
State mental hospitals and the process of
deinstitutionalization

In the previous chapter as we started to describe mental disorders, mention was made about the *early views* related to psychopathology. Partly because of the powerful influence of the church, and partly because of pure ignorance, in the most part, mental illness was attributed to supernatural forces. Those afflicted with mental illness were viewed as sinners who were possessed by demonic spirits. It was believed that the punishment meted out by the gods resulted in abnormal behaviors. This belief prevailed throughout the course of the history of Western societies through the Middle Ages. Mentally ill people were isolated from mainstream society, and were "warehoused" in rural areas in asylums. People often feared them because their behavior was bizarre and unpredictable. They were treated as if they were dangerous criminals, and kept under horrendous circumstances. They were shackled, minimally fed, and were housed in dark unsanitary conditions. They were often subjected to physical punishments and torture. Frequently they were used as means of entertainment for the general public. People came to observe their unusual behaviors as a form of fun and leisure activity. Exorcism was used at times in an attempt to free these sick individuals from demonic possession.

In the eighteenth century some positive changes started to emerge. In France the pioneering efforts of Jean-Baptiste Pussin and Philippe Pinel led to the beginnings of *moral therapy.* Pussin and Pinel were progressive thinkers who professed that mentally abnormal people were suffering from an illness, and were not to be blamed for their unfortunate condition. They insisted that these sick individuals deserved to be treated with respect in sanitary environments. This humane philosophy of treatment resulted in the unchaining of inmates, and the elimination of punitive treatments. In fact many inmates were released from these asylums. The success of compassionate treatment led to similar approaches in England and Italy. In the United States in the early part of the nineteenth century Benjamin Rush and Dorothea Dix have been credited for their work related to the social and medical needs of mentally ill patients. The establishment of mental hospitals and attempts at the medical management of mental abnormalities in the United States are largely attributable to the insights and initiatives of Rush and Dix.

While moral therapy, which included kind words, understanding, empathy, clean and friendly physical environment, better nutrition, exposure to sunlight, and occupational therapy, helped in the successful recovery of many patients, it was not effective in the treatment of severely disturbed individuals. Consequently this approach to treatment slowly faded away. Conditions in mental hospitals gradually deteriorated, and there was little hope left for the severely ill. Custodial care was substandard, unsanitary and neglectful. This situation prevailed through the middle of the twentieth century.

Several other developments in the late nineteenth and early twentieth centuries had significant impact on the management of mental illness. The German psychiatrist, Emil Kraepelin is known for his very influential work on the classification of mental illnesses. His elaboration on specific symptoms and treatment responsiveness, including the cognitive and behavioral effects of a variety of drugs, paved the way for a more scientific understanding of psychiatric disorders. Lightner Witmer also played an important part in history. A psychologist, and a student of Wilhelm Wundt (the founder of experimental psychology), Witmer established in 1896 the world's first clinic devoted exclusively for the treatment of mental disorders. In 1908 he founded the first residential school to serve children with emotional problems and retarded cognitive development. In France in the late nineteenth century, the research work of Jean-Martin Charcot shed further light on the etiology of mental illnesses. He lectured extensively on the physiological and psychological aspects of abnormal behavior, and the use of hypnosis in clinical practice. His findings were highly influential in the foundation of psychoanalysis, which was further developed by Sigmund Freud (Hergenhahn, 2009).

In our country the state-run mental hospitals were found in rural areas, spread over many acres of land. They were designed for the long term hospitalization of many thousands of patients. The expectation was that these patients would never be released, because their condition was chronic, and there were no known effective remedies at that time. These hospitals were self-contained communities equipped with medical facilities, dining facilities, recreational centers, schools, occupational areas, houses of worship, and facilities for outdoor activities. Unfortunately the quality of care offered to patients significantly declined over the years. Over time abuse of patients became rampant.

Eventually the deteriorating conditions in state mental institutions throughout the United States caught public attention. In the 1950's a new trend started to develop. Prolonged custodial care was viewed as counterproductive to the healing process. Patients became dependent on these institutions, and lost their ability to function on their own even in the most elementary aspects of daily living. Consequently plans were formulated to reintegrate as many patients as possible into the community. This process, know as *deinstitutionalization* was facilitated by the introduction of newly developed drugs which aimed to control major symptoms associated with schizophrenia, such as delusions and hallucinations.

The alternative to institutional care was known as *community-based care*. Many *community mental health centers* were erected. These centers were designed to offer comprehensive services. Patients received individual and group psychotherapy by qualified psychologists. Psychiatrists and nurses provided medication management. When necessary, patients were referred to other medical specialists. Day care programs included recreational activities and arrangements for vocational training. Productive and paid employment was offered to qualified clients. Supervised housing facilities were also available through the auspices of these mental health centers. The philosophy and purpose of this movement was to create an easy transition from years of hospitalization to independent community living. This program was partially successful and is still in existence today. Over the past decades many state mental hospitals were permanently closed down. Others are still open today, but with a much-reduced census. Unfortunately some chronic patients need the continued support of hospitals.

SECTION 7.2:
OUTPATIENT AND INPATIENT TREATMENT

The following topics are discussed in this section:
Details related to outpatient and inpatient treatment
Patients' right to dispute the need for hospitalization
Conditions which require chronic inpatient/institutional
care

The treatment of psychological disorders takes place in one of two settings: *outpatient* or *inpatient*. Generally speaking, outpatient treatment is intended for those patients who are not deemed dangerous to self or to others, who are in a relatively stable condition, able to ambulate, and are sufficiently compliant with treatment recommendations. Outpatient treatment is offered in hospital based psychiatric outpatient departments, free-standing psychiatric clinics, and in offices of private mental health practitioners. Outpatient treatment may be in the form of individual, group, couple or family psychotherapy, depending on the need of clients. Medication and electroconvulsive (ECT) therapy is prescribed for the management of more serious conditions. Outpatient visits for psychotherapy are ordinarily scheduled on a weekly basis; and for medication and ECT management on a four to six week basis.

Inpatient treatment may be short or long term. The purpose of short-term treatment is round-the-clock observation, determination of dangerousness to self or to others, and discontinuation and change of medication types and dosages in a controlled and safe professional environment. Patients often resist inpatient hospitalization, especially when they are in an agitated state, lacking insight and good judgment. Police intervention may be needed to facilitate the transportation of patients to the psychiatric emergency room and hospital. The recommendation of two physicians is needed in order to hospitalize a patient against his/her will. Following a brief hospital stay, patients have the right for free legal representation, and court appearance, where a judge decides if continued hospitalization is warranted.

The judge's decision is based upon the professional opinion of the treating psychiatrist, the patient's compliance with treatment efforts in the hospital, the potential family or social support for the patient in the community, and the patient's reasons for wanting to leave the hospital. While in the hospital, patients receive a thorough diagnostic work-up, medications, electroshock therapy (when indicated), as well as individual and group therapy. Art therapy, movement therapy, and recreational opportunities are also provided. Patients' relatives and significant others are offered consultation with the patient's treating psychiatrist and other members of the treatment team (i.e. social workers, psychologists). Upon the stabilization of the patient's condition, social workers make arrangements for outpatient follow-up care. Recommendations related to the management of patients at home are given to families.

Patients with serious and treatment-resistant conditions may need long-term hospitalization. State psychiatric and developmental centers are equipped for long-term stay. Patients who require chronic inpatient care usually suffer from certain types of schizophrenia or severe mood disorders. Severe cases of dementia, mental retardation, and traumatic brain injury also require institutional care.

SECTION 7.3:
PROVIDERS OF MENTAL HEALTH SERVICES

The following topics are discussed in this section:
Educational requirements of mental health professionals
Specialization of mental health professionals

It is wise for patients to become "educated consumers" of mental health services. To this end I will list the types of mental health professionals who provide services to the public.

Clinical psychologists possess a doctoral degree in psychology. In the United States of America there are three types of recognized doctoral degrees: Doctor of Philosophy (Ph.D.), Doctor of Psychology (Psy.D.), and Doctor of Education (Ed.D.). Passing a licensing examination is required in order to practice independently. Clinical psychologists diagnose and treat mental disorders using psychological techniques. Some clinical psychologists specialize in the treatment of children and adolescents. They also administer psychological tests. In some states (currently New Mexico and Louisiana), with additional training, clinical psychologists are allowed to prescribe psychiatric medications.

Counseling psychologists also possess doctoral degrees in psychology and need to pass a licensing examination. Their functions are very similar to those of clinical psychologists. They usually treat patients with less severe mental disorders. They often work in the counseling centers of college campuses, where they help students who have problems with academic adjustment and career choices. They also work with new immigrants who have acculturation and other social adjustment difficulties.

Neuropsychologists specialize in the diagnosis and treatment of organic brain disorders, including learning disabilities.

School psychologists with master or doctoral degrees work in public or private schools. They diagnose emotional problems and learning disabilities related to academic performance of pupils. When needed they treat or make referrals for treatment.

Psychiatrists are physicians who have earned the degree of Doctor of Medicine (M.D.). They need to complete a psychiatric residency program of three to five years duration in a teaching hospital. Some psychiatrists specialize in the treatment of children, older adults (geriatrics) and patients with addictive disorders. In today's managed health care environment most psychiatrists diagnose and treat mental illnesses. Their treatment intervention most often involve the use of psychiatric drugs. Only a minority of psychiatrists engage their patients in psychotherapy.

Psychoanalysts are mental health professionals who possess advanced degrees (e.g. Ph.D., M.D., M.S.W.), and who also have received additional training and experience in the techniques of psychoanalysis.

Psychiatric social workers have received a master's degree (M.S.W.) or doctoral degree (D.S.W.) in social work. They are knowledgeable in the specific services which social agencies provide for the mentally ill. They help patients gain access to financial support, treatment and housing. Many social workers also practice marital and family therapy. Some, with specialized post-graduate training, also provide individual and group psychotherapy. Clinical social workers must have six years of supervised training and must pass a licensing examination.

Counselors ordinarily have earned a master's degree (M.A. or M.S.) They often work with patients who have a substance abuse problem. They may perform vocational evaluations, assist in special educational testing, and perform family and marital counseling. Mental health counselors and marriage and family counselors must be licensed.

When looking for psychological/psychiatric services, it is very important to be familiar with the educational qualifications of service providers. The law requires providers to be licensed or certified in their specializations.

SECTION 7.4:
PSYCHOTHERAPY

The following topics are addressed in this section:
The definition of psychotherapy
Description and origins of therapeutic orientations
The process of psychological therapy
The requirements for successful therapeutic outcomes

We often hear the word "therapy". But what exactly is psychotherapy? What is the difference between "just talking and listening" and formal therapy? What are the origins of psychotherapy? Why are there so many kinds of therapy? Are psychological treatments effective? Who can benefit from therapy? How does the psychotherapeutic process work? What are the characteristics of an experienced and ethical therapist? How do we select a competent psychotherapist? These are some of the questions we will explore in the following pages.

The definition can be expressed in simple terms. The use of verbal means to help an individual with a mental disturbance is called psychotherapy. Formal therapy is very different from "just talking and listening". Professional psychotherapists use methods which are grounded in established theories and well documented psychological principles. In order to fully appreciate the meaning of the most frequently used therapies, we need to briefly review the theories in which these therapies have been rooted.

Psychodynamic therapy: While there were many early philosophers, scientists, physicians and other thinkers who speculated about the composition of the mind and abnormalities of behavior, it was Sigmund Freud (1856-1939) who developed the first organized psychological model of abnormal behavior. It is called the *psychodynamic model*. Freud and his followers believed that the origins of psychological *disturbances* can be traced back to unresolved childhood conflicts. According to this model the mind has three distinct layers: the *conscious*, the *preconscious*, and the *unconscious*. Wakeful awareness is the domain of the conscious layer. The conscious mind facilitates our proper orientation to self (understanding who we are), space (understanding where we are), and time (knowing the time of day, the date and season of year). The preconscious layer contains memories which are easily accessible as the need arises. For example, names of our family members and our date of birth can be easily retrieved from preconscious memory. The unconscious is the largest layer. It contains our primitive aggressive and sexual instincts, hurtful life experiences, and wishes which may cause us severe anxiety. According to the psychodynamic model these instincts and thoughts need to be kept out of conscious awareness because they may give rise to socially unacceptable behaviors or cause emotional disturbances. We tend to *repress* (push out of awareness) thoughts and urges which may lead to socially improper expression. Repression protects us from anxiety resulting from dwelling upon sexual and aggressive instincts. Exposure to negative experiences such as parental abuse, neglect, or loss of significant family members in the course of our formative years can have an untoward effect on our emotions and behavior as adults.

Psychoanalysis aims to uncover unconscious conflicts and trauma and thereby help patients achieve improved levels of adjustment with minimal anxiety. The two main techniques used to delve into the unconscious are *free association* and *dream analysis*. Free association involves verbalizing all thoughts as they come to mind, without any inhibitions. The aim is to explore hidden impulses and conflicts, bring them to the conscious level, and then resolve them in a rational fashion. According to psychodynamic theory as we sleep, our psychological defenses are weakened, and many of our socially unacceptable wishes and fantasies are spilled into our dreams. Hence reviewing the meaning of our dream content with the psychoanalyst may facilitate a better understanding of our unconscious processes. Traditional psychoanalysis is a lengthy and expensive method of therapy, often lasting for several years. The relatively recent and modern psychodynamic approaches are more pragmatic, briefer and more directly focused on the acquisition of adaptive behaviors useful in daily life.

Behavior therapy: The roots of behavior therapy date back to the early 1900's, when the school of thought known as "behaviorism" was established by famous psychologists such as John Watson (1878-1958) and Burrhus Skinner (1904-1990). These pioneering thinkers insisted that psychology should become a "scientific" discipline and subscribe to the rigorous methods of research which are followed by the "hard" sciences, such as physics and chemistry. They proposed that psychology should only concern itself with "observable" behaviors. They vehemently opposed psychodynamic constructs such as "id, ego and superego". They rejected the phenomenon of the "unconscious", and all other unobservable "mentalistic" ideas. They claimed that the fundamental requirements of the scientific method is the ability to objectively observe and measure. The study of the relationship between environmental stimulation and consequent behavior was at the heart of behavioral psychology. Learning, and the effects of rewards and punishment on behavior took a central focus in research.

The Russian physician and physiologist, Ivan Pavlov (1849-1936) was also very influential in promoting the scientific stature of psychology. His findings paved the way to our understanding of "learning by association". Pavlov demonstrated that naturally occurring responses, such as salivation when food is introduced in our mouth, may be elicited by those events which precede the experience of tasting food. Let us consider the following example. Suppose you regularly visit your grandmother for dinner every Friday evening. You sit in her dining room hungry, waiting for the delicious chicken soup to be served. As you are eagerly waiting, you start hearing the clanging of pots and plates in the kitchen nearby. All of a sudden you begin to feel that your mouth is getting wet with saliva. What is the reason for this? It has to do with conditioning. Upon your previous visits to your grandmother, the clanging sounds originating in the kitchen was followed by the serving of chicken soup. Hence you learned to *associate* the sound with the taste of the soup. Many emotional responses, such as fear and sexual excitement, can also be learned by this associative process.

The techniques involved in behavior therapy rely upon a variety of learning principles. The aim is to help patients acquire modes of behavior which will help them improve the quality of their lives. The assumption is that all behaviors are the result of learning experiences. Therefore in order to learn more adaptive behaviors, the patient needs to do two things: unlearn those patterns of behavior which cause problems, and then learn new productive ways of interacting with the environment (i.e. people and situations) Unlike psychoanalysis, behavior therapy focuses on the present, and deals with targeted maladaptive behaviors which need to be changed in a relatively short period of time. Issues related to feelings and emotions are deemphasized.

Some of the more frequently used behavioral techniques used in clinical practice include *behavior modification, gradual exposure, systematic desensitization,* and *modeling.* Behavior modification involves the systematic use of reinforcements (rewards) and punishments in an attempt to eradicate unwanted behaviors (e.g. temper tantrums) and encourage adaptive (desirable) modes of behaving. Severe fears and phobias are treated using gradual exposure and systematic desensitization. Patients are progressively exposed to objects and situations which they have been fearfully avoiding. They are also taught to use relaxation exercises when faced with fear evoking events. Modeling involves asking patients to repeatedly imitate new coping strategies demonstrated by a therapist with the aim of permanently learning important target behaviors such as improved communication or social skills.

Cognitive therapy: Our way of thinking and the manner in which we conceptualize and evaluate potentially stressful events greatly affect our emotional reactions and our ability to cope with the challenges posed in daily life. The aim of cognitive therapy is to help patients realize that attitudes, beliefs, misinformation, and preconceptions related to difficulties in life may result in anxiety and depression. Oftentimes our interpretations and expectations related to misfortunes are more debilitating than the troubling events themselves. Albert Ellis (1913-2007) is probably the best-known psychologist in the area of *rational emotive behavior therapy*. It was his belief that negative feelings are directly related to irrational and self-defeating beliefs. For example some people may strongly believe that they must be loved and accepted by all those who they find important in their lives. Ellis and other cognitive therapists agree that it is certainly nice to be loved and accepted, but that it is a mistake to believe that this love and acceptance is crucial for survival. It is more adaptive to believe that the support of others is beneficial, but what is most important in life is self-reliance, and dependence one one's own strengths and skills.

Aaron Beck is a famous and influential cognitive psychiatrist. Beck and his colleagues proposed that people often commit errors in their thinking processes. These errors are called *cognitive distortions*. These distortions may in turn result in symptoms of anxiety and depression. Magnification (catastrophizing) of relatively insignificant problems, minimization of one's achievements, jumping to illogical negative conclusions are examples of cognitive distortions. Beck's cognitive therapy aims at the identification and alteration of thinking errors, thereby helping clients view themselves and the world around them in a more realistic and adaptive fashion.

Cognitive-behavior therapy: Most behavior therapy practitioners use a combined cognitive and behavioral approach to achieve realistic and adaptive modes of coping with problems and reaching goals in life. The aim of therapy is to effect changes in self-defeating observable behaviors and underlying defective thought patterns. Clients' openness to change and willingness to learn new approaches and solutions to problems are essential for positive outcomes in behavior and cognitive therapies.

Humanistic therapy: Abraham Maslow (1908-1970) and Carl Rogers (1902-1987) are probably the most prominent humanistic psychologists. The movement, called *humanistic psychology*, gained popularity in the 1950's. In contrast to the teachings of behavioral and psychodynamic thinkers, humanistic psychologists posited that free will, conscious choices, and goal-oriented endeavors are central to human existence. Obstructive forces, such as oppressive parenting methods or destructive relationships, which prevent people from following the road to their life goals and desires may result in mental illness. Self-knowledge, the awareness of subjective strengths, weaknesses, tastes, and wishes were considered important in managing one's life successfully. Fulfilling an individual's potentials in a meaningful and purposeful manner was viewed as essential requirements for healthy adjustment and happiness. Clients are encouraged to engage in self-exploration, and to accept their true selves, without any pretenses. The focus of humanistic or *client-centered* therapy is the achievement of comfortable adjustment and the exercise of free will. The emphasis is on the "here and now" and finding avenues to maximally use the individual's potentials in order to achieve total fulfillment of life goals and aspirations, also known as *self-actualization*. Efforts are made to make clients feel safe and unconditionally accepted in the therapeutic process. The therapist's role is that of a facilitator, allowing the client to set the tone and content of the therapy sessions.

Gestalt therapy is another form of humanistic therapy. The originator of this approach was Fritz Perls (1893-1970). This method of treatment is based on the ideas proposed by the Gestalt school of psychology. According to this school of thought the human brain is capable to organize our percepts into meaningful experiences as opposed to bits and pieces of events which we see or hear. Gestalt therapists aim to integrate the conflicting parts of the client's personality. They encourage clients to get in touch with their innermost feelings, bring them into consciousness, and express all conflicting sensations as they presently experience them. Role-playing exercises and imaginary conflict resolution techniques are used in this process. The ultimate aim is free, uninhibited expression of feelings.

Eclectic therapy: The solutions to patients' problems cannot always be fit into a single theoretical framework. Consequently therapists often use a variety of therapeutic approaches to help patients gain insight, learn better coping skills and improve their adjustment to ever-changing environmental demands. The eclectic approach allows for flexibility as therapists apply the most suitable philosophies and methods in treating their clients.

Group therapy: Certain problems and conditions are best treated in a group setting. In this process the therapist seats about seven patients in a circle to address symptoms and problems which they have in common. Examples of topics for discussion are ways to alleviate symptoms of anxiety and depression. Issues related to childrearing, divorce, bereavement, substance abuse, anger management, and acculturation may also be addressed in group therapy. This modality is especially useful for clients who need social support and feedback related to their social skills. Listening and learning from each other's experiences and coping skills can be very valuable in the therapeutic process. The therapist usually assumes a facilitative role, and assures mutual respect, and confidentiality among group members. Group members are encouraged to listen and participate in discussions without dominating the group process. Group therapy may be recommended as an adjunctive method to individual psychotherapy. Not all clients are willing to partake in group therapy. People may feel more comfortable on a one-on-one setting as they disclose their problems and deep-seated feelings.

Couple therapy: Married or unmarried couples with relationship problems may be advised to participate in couple therapy. The goal of this approach is to give couples the opportunity to discuss their difficulties objectively in a non-judgmental setting in front of a trained professional. Examples of topics for discussion are issues related to fidelity, communication, gender roles, and jealousy. Individual psychotherapy may be recommended prior to the initiation of couple therapy.

Family therapy: Damaged family lives are often best addressed in family therapy. Behavioral dynamics within the family are analyzed by specially trained family therapists. Common problems include scapegoating, excessive dominance, control, role relationships, and conflicts related to adolescent rebellion. The therapist facilitates the flow of communication during the session, and may offer ideas for conflict resolution. At times more than one family participates in the therapy session. *Multifamily therapy* is indicated for families which share similar problems. In this setting family members discuss stressors and conflicts which are of mutual interest. The advantages here are opportunities for feedback, and learning from the mistakes and successes of others.

Psychoeducational therapy: Many of us find psychopathology an obscure phenomenon. We may not understand the causes, symptoms, and mechanisms of abnormal behavior. Some people think that bizarre conduct is voluntary, and that the person manifesting "strange" symptoms can simply stop behaving "strangely" if he only "wanted to". The purpose of psychoeducational therapy is to educate the afflicted person and his/her significant others about the biological, psychological and social aspects of mental illness. Pharmacological and psychological treatment modalitiess are also discussed.

Uninformed individuals are often puzzled about the value and processes involved in psychological therapies. Research findings tell us that psychotherapy is a very beneficial treatment modality (Smith, Glass, & Miller, 1980). It is important to "shop around" for the right therapist in order to maximally benefit from treatment. Prospective clients may wish to select therapists with whom they can easily "connect". Easy connection may depend on the ethnicity, religion, sex, age, personality, and theoretical orientation of the professional person. It must be remembered that therapy is a lengthy process, with weekly one-hour sessions often going on for many months; hence "getting along" with the therapist, and feeling comfortable in the office is of paramount importance. It is advisable to have an informative discussion with therapists prior to committing for treatment. Prospective clients need to be "educated consumers of mental health services". Introductory topics for discussion should include matters related to the therapeutic process, limits of confidentiality, frequency of visits, anticipated results, and costs.

Psychotherapy is not a passive undertaking. Regardless of the theoretical orientation used, the client needs to be an active participant in the process. Therapists may even give "homework assignments" or "behavioral prescriptions" to clients to be completed between therapy sessions. In general, psychotherapy has two purposes: stress release, and education. Stress release results in emotional comfort, and education promotes new coping strategies and skills required for improved adjustment and continued success in many facets of life. The effectiveness of therapy is in many ways dependent upon the client's commitment to the therapeutic procedures. Psychotherapy in many ways is a learning process, with the ultimate aim of effectuating emotional, cognitive, and behavioral changes. Clients must be willing to abandon maladaptive behaviors, and acquire new ways of dealing with a variety of challenges in their lives. This process of change is often hard and frustrating. It is certainly not easy to alter well-established patterns of behavior, or to give up chronic habits. Persistent determination, work, and self-evaluation on the part of the client is an absolute necessity for changes to take hold.

SECTION 7.5:
PSYCHOPHARMACOLOGICAL TREATMENT

The following topics are discussed in this section:
Brief history of psychopharmacology
Brief neuroanatomy, and neurophysiology related to drug
actions
Review of classes of psychoactive drugs and their mecha-
nism of action

There is a long history leading to the beginnings of the use of psychoactive drugs. Historically drugs have been used for both recreational and therapeutic purposes. The same is true in today's world. In early times drugs played a major role in religious rituals. People took drugs in their attempts to facilitate spiritual experiences and to reach and communicate with heavenly forces. The writings of ancient physicians are testimony to the use of medicines for the treatment of mental disorders. Opium, alcohol, hemp, and a variety of herbs and potions have been used by the Babylonians, Egyptians, Romans, Hindus, Chinese, and Greeks. (Hergenhahn, 500r). Emil Kraepelin, the famous German psychiatrist is believed to be the first scientist to systematically study the behavioral effects of drugs. In 1892 He coined the term "pharmacopsychology", which we now call *psychopharmacology* (the study of the use of medications which affect mental functioning and behavior). He also studied the effects of addictive substances such as alcohol, morphine and caffeine, on a variety of intellectual functions (Schmied, Steinberg, & Sykes, 2006).

Mental illness, as it is understood today, has a biological, psychological, and social component. The actual amount of "weight" or influence of any one of these components is variable. As it was discussed in a previous section of this book, some mental illnesses have a strong biological component; others may be weighed more heavily on the psychological or social factors. In cases such as in bipolar illness and schizophrenia where biological factors play an important role, psychopharmacological intervention is usually a necessary part of treatment.

The biochemistry and physiology of the nervous system is quite complex. In order to gain some understanding of the mechanism of drug actions, the reader must be familiar with some very basic neurological terms and concepts. In an earlier section of this book I made references to some basic aspects of the nervous system. Here I will review this information again in some more detail. Cells found in the nervous system are called *neurons* (please refer to the diagram of the neuron for an easier conceptualization of this material). Neurons are physically supported (held together) by *glial cells*. These supporting cells also provide nourishment to neurons, remove their toxic waste products, and assist in neural communication. There are several types of neurons: *Sensory (afferent) neurons* conduct information from sensory organs (e.g. eyes, ears), muscles, and inner organs to the spinal cord and brain. *Motor (efferent) neurons* carry information from the *central nervous system* (brain and spinal cord) to muscles and glands. As these messages arrive, muscles will move, and glands will secrete hormones, which are necessary for proper bodily functions. *Interneurons (associative neurons)* connect one neuron to another, functionally similar to an electrical extension cord. These are the most commonly found neurons in the nervous system. Interneurons in the brain are responsible for many of our intellectual processes, such as conceptualizing, problem solving and planning. Neurons are designed to transmit messages in the form of electrical impulses. Neurons have specific anatomical areas serving unique functions in the process of information transmission. The *soma* or *cell body* contains structures (e.g. mitochondria) whose function is to keep the cell alive. The cell nucleus, including genetic material is also found in the cell body. Neurons are enclosed by a *cell membrane*. This membrane sets the boundary between the existing biochemical environment inside and outside the neuron. The projections arising from the cell body are called *dendrites*. The function of dendrites is to receive information from neighboring cells. The *axon* is a long extension structure connected to the soma, which conducts impulses going out to other neurons. Many axons have an insulating layer of a fatty substance called *myelin sheath* along their length. The myelin is produced by the glial cells. At certain points along the axon there are tiny gaps in the myelin casing. These gaps are called *nodes of Ranvier*. Myelinization results in faster neural transmission. The electrical impulse seems to hop very rapidly between these gaps all the way to the end of the axon. Depending on their location in the body, the size of axons vary in both length and diameter. The *synaptic vesicles* (*terminal buttons*) located at the end points of axons, contain chemical substances called *neurotransmitters*. These neurotransmitters are produced in the cell body. There are many kinds of neurotransmitters. There is no physical connection among neurons. The tiny gap which separates neurons from one another is called the *synapse*. Neurotransmitters act as "biochemical bridges" to facilitate the conduction of impulses between adjacent neurons. As the neural message reaches the end of the axon, the terminal buttons spill their neurotransmitter content into the synapse. These chemicals in turn travel across the synapse and lock onto the receptor sites located on the dendrites of the adjacent receiving neuron. Receptor sites are designed to accept only specific types of neurotransmitter molecules; this mechanism is similar to the way a key fits into a lock.

Neural communication therefore has both electrical and chemical properties. It is an *electrochemical* event. Depending on their chemical structure, the action of neurotransmitters on receiving (*postsynaptic*) neurons may result in *excitation* (increased activity) or *inhibition* (decreased activity) of further neural transmission. Optimal neural functioning depends upon the correct balance between excitation and inhibition. Following the passage of information to the receiving neuron, the residual neurotransmitters must be removed from the synapse in order to prevent excessive continuous stimulation of the postsynaptic neurons. The nervous system has three natural mechanisms to prevent excessive neural stimulation: *reuptake*, *enzymatic action*, and *neuromodulator action*. In the reuptake process residual neurotransmitters are reabsorbed by their vesicles for future use in the conduction of impulses. In the process of enzymatic action, enzymes (organic catalysts) break down left-over neurotransmitters in the synapse in order to prepare them for elimination. Neuromodulators are biochemical compounds which can influence (decrease) the sensitivity of postsynaptic neurons to incoming neurotransmitters.

Now that we have reviewed these very basic concepts about the nervous system, we are armed with sufficient knowledge to appreciate on a fundamental level the biochemistry and physiology of some mental illnesses, and the manner in which psychopharmacological agents (medications) work. The biological abnormalities associated with mental illnesses fall into two main categories: structural and/or functional damage. Structural damage means insult to brain tissue, which may result from trauma associated with car accidents or gunshot wounds or other incidents. Structural brain damage may also result from chromosomal abnormalities; a familiar example is Down's syndrome, involving various levels of mental retardation. Benign or malignant brain tumors, strokes, and aneurysms (bursting of weak blood vessels) also cause tissue damage. Structural damage certainly may negatively affect the physiological and biochemical aspects of brain functioning. In most cases functional damage is related to biochemical (neurotransmitter) imbalance in the brain, and irregularities in neural conduction. Medications intended to reduce or alleviate symptoms of mental illness are targeted to restore biochemical (neurotransmitter) balance, and/or rectify the physiological process of neural impulse transmission.

In order to appreciate the mechanism of psychoactive drug action, we need to reflect back upon the introductory paragraphs of this section. The targeted anatomical area is the synapse, because this is the site of important biochemical activity.

Medications may effectuate changes in the brain in any one or more of the following ways:
- Affecting (increasing or decreasing) the synthesis (production) of neurotransmitters
- Preventing the storage of neurotransmitters in the synaptic vesicles (terminal buttons)

- Stimulating or inhibiting the release of neurotransmitters from the synaptic vesicles
- Stimulating or blocking postsynaptic receptors (receptors on receiving neurons)
- Inhibiting neurotransmitter degradation (breaking down by enzymes)
- Blocking reuptake (reabsorption into terminal buttons) of neurotransmitters

(Meyer & Quenzer, 2005)

Psychopharmacological intervention is usually indicated in the treatment of the following psychological disorders: affective (mood) disorders, anxiety disorders, and psychotic disorders. I will now discuss classes of medications used. Specific names, uses, and side effects of medications belonging to these classes are listed in the appendix.

The oldest antidepressant medications are the *monoamine oxidase inhibitors (MAOIs)*. These drugs target the enzyme monoamine oxidase, which metabolizes (breaks down) neurotransmitters (serotonin and norepinephrine) in presynaptic vesicles, hence slowing down neural transmission. These antidepressant drugs inhibit this enzymatic action, and thereby improve neural transmission. The *tricyclic antidepressants* inhibit the reuptake of neurotransmitters into the presynaptic vesicles, thereby increasing the duration of transmitter activity at the synaptic junctures. The *selective serotonin reuptake inhibitors* (SSRIs) inhibit the reuptake of the neurotransmitter serotonin, which plays a significant biochemical role in mood regulation. *Lithium carbonate* is usually the drug of choice for the treatment of bipolar disorder. It elevates brain *tryptophan*, an amino acid essential to the synthesis of serotonin. It also reduces the stimulating effects of *catecholamines* (excitatory neurotransmitters). In addition to lithium other classes of medications also have been prescribed for the treatment of bipolar disorder. These include anticonvulsants, antipsychotics, anxiolytics, and antidepressants (Kelsey, Newport, & Nemeroff, 2006).

The oldest *anxiolytic* (anxiety reducing) drugs are the *barbiturates*.

They relieve feelings of worry and tension, and are helpful in tolerating stress. They also have a *hypnotic* (sleep inducing) effect at higher doses. Barbiturates increase the effects of gamma-aminobutyric acid (GABA), which is an inhibitory neurotransmitter; this results in a generalized slowing of neuronal excitability in the brain. These drugs are highly addictive and have serious side effects, hence over the years their medical use has declined.

The *benzodiazepines* are powerful anxiolytic agents. Their mechanism of action is similar to that of the barbiturates, in that they also act on GABA. The addictive and side effects of these drugs are less serious and rarely lethal; hence psychiatrists prescribe them more readily.

An example of a so-called *second-generation* anxiolytic medication is *buspirone*. Among physicians this is a preferred drug because both side effects (e.g. sedation and confusion) and recreational use are minimal. Furthermore, buspirone is also effective in the treatment of depression, which commonly occurs in patients suffering from anxiety. The therapeutic effect of the drug however, is not as rapid as that of the other classes of anxiolytics. Pharmacologically buspirone increases serotonin availability at neural receptor sites in various brain areas (Meyer & Quenzer, 2005).

Antipsychotic drugs are also called *neuroleptics*. They reduce psychomotor activity and emotionality, symptoms which are characteristic of psychotic disorders, especially schizophrenia. The traditional neuroleptics include the *phenothiazines* and *butyrophenones*. The mechanism of action of these drugs involves the reduction of neural transmission mediated by the neurotransmitter *dopamine*. The drugs may either block dopamine receptors, or inhibit the release of dopamine from the terminal vesicles. Traditional neuroleptics target the *positive symptoms* of schizophrenia, such as hallucinations, delusions, and disorganized speech. Side effects can be very serious, irreversible, and lethal. The *atypical antipsychotics* are often considered the drugs of choice because they produce less side effects (movement disorders), and reduce both positive and negative symptoms (e.g. deficits in emotional responsiveness, loss of motivation and initiative, and social withdrawal).

There are many psychoactive medications available for the treatment of mental disorders. The reason for this large selection is that individual reactions to these drugs vary greatly in the population. Persistent, dangerous and uncomfortable side effects greatly contribute to poor compliance. Consequently drug manufacturers try to synthesize compounds which are more tolerable and pose less health risks. Appendix XVIII lists the most commonly used drugs and their side effects.

SECTION 7.6:
MISCELLANEOUS BIOLOGICAL THERAPIES

The following topics are discussed in this section:
Description of electroconvulsive therapy
Description of transcranial magnetic stimulation
Description of light therapy
Description of deep brain stimulation

In addition to psychotherapy and pharmacological therapy there are several less well-known methods used to treat mental illness.

Electroconvulsive therapy (ECT): The therapeutic utility of ECT was discovered accidentally by a Hungarian psychiatrist in the early 1900's. He noted that a number of his patients showed an improvement in mood following a seizure attack. This observation led to the idea of artificial seizure inducement for the treatment of depression. The procedure involves the passing of a mild and brief electrical current through the head. It is believed that ECT acts upon several important neurotransmitters in the brain. The patient is anesthetized, and is given muscle relaxants and oxygen to prevent convulsions and to maintain respiration. ECT is usually administered three times a week for a three-week period. The procedure is offered to patients who are non-responsive to other treatment modalities, or who cannot tolerate medication side effects. Pregnant women, elderly and medically ill patients are good candidates for this treatment modality because the side effects are minimal. Temporary memory loss is the most prominent side effect (Meyer & Quenzer, 2005).

Transcranial magnetic stimulation (TMS): This is a relatively new technique. The procedure involves magnetic induction through the skull, which then results in a weak and localized electric current in the brain, causing alterations in neural activity. Patients suffering from depression can benefit from this treatment. The procedure is painless, requiring no anesthesia or muscle relaxants. Side effects are minimal (Meyer & Quenzer, 2005).

Light therapy (phototherapy): Seasonal affective disorder is a type of depression which most often occurs in the winter months. Exposure to artificial bright white light (light boxes) for several hours a day results in symptomatic relief. Extra exposure to light affects the regulation of the hormone melatonin, which according to some theories may be associated with this depressive disorder. Light therapy should not be attempted without the recommendation of a psychiatrist.

Deep brain stimulation (DBS): This is an innovative treatment of last resort for depressed patients who do not benefit from more conventional methods. Surgery is required to implant electrodes into the brain, and to implant pulse generators into the chest. Over a period of several months the pulse generators will send electrical signals to stimulate the brain. The concept and mechanism is similar to that of a pacemaker.

CHAPTER EIGHT:

Mental Health and the Law

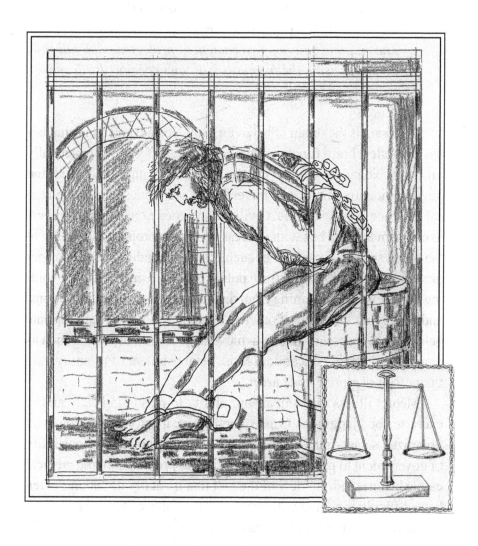

"He threatens many that hath injured one."
BEN JOHNSON

SECTION 8.1:
INTRODUCTION

The following topics are discussed this section:
The responsibility of government to protect society
The responsibility of government to protect mentally ill individuals using the framework of laws specifically drawn for this purpose

The brain is the organ of behavior. Both normal and abnormal behaviors reflect brain function. Our behavior is affected by genetically inherited biological determinants, current ongoing anatomical and physiological functions, and material learned from social and physical environmental exposure. Civilized societies expect their members to conform to basic behaviors necessary for the proper functioning of the social system. Examples of such essential conduct include proper dressing habits (refraining from public nudity), using toilets for voiding human waste, refraining from dangerous and threatening actions, and respecting the rights of others. Adherence to socially appropriate behaviors is necessary for the achievement of ordinary goals such as reaching a certain educational level, establishment of a family, and the pursuit of a preferred career.

Mental illness may impair our ability to reason logically and to exercise good judgment. Consequently our capacity to function in an organized society may become compromised. It is the responsibility of government to protect its citizens, and to provide humane medical care when needed. In view of the fact that mentally ill patients often have difficulties coping with the demands of daily life, and may pose a danger to themselves or others as a consequence of their psychiatric disorder, it is the responsibility of the government to provide protection. Governments have introduced laws in order to effectively carry out this protective responsibility. Protection also includes the preservation of fundamental human rights. Both healthy and mentally sick individuals have legally guaranteed rights.

Given the fact that mentally ill individuals often lack insight, and may be unable to appreciate the nature and severity of their condition, and are frequently unable to procure the help they need, or may not understand the psychiatric treatments they require, the law provides special guidelines associated with the management of these persons. The laws discussed in this chapter either pertain to the United States (federal) or exclusively to New York State. These laws may be rooted in the constitutions, or they may be statutes enacted by the legislature, or rules of court adopted by the judiciary, or decisions made by courts (case law) (Behnke, Perlin, & Bernstein, 2003). Other states within the United States of America have similar laws. Civilized countries around the world likewise have laws exclusively addressing the needs and protection of mentally ill persons.

SECTION 8.2:
PRIVACY, CONFIDENTIALITY, AND
TESTIMONIAL PRIVILEGE

The following topics are discussed in this section:
The meaning of privacy, confidentiality and testimonial
privilege in the context of mental health services
The limits of confidentiality and testimonial privilege in
doctor-patient relationships
The right to informed consent to psychiatric treatment
Time limitations for malpractice lawsuits against physi-
cians and psychologists

Privacy is a fundamental civil right. It has to do with autonomy, or self-determination as we conduct our lives in society. Privacy allows us to live our lives in accordance with the choices me make. For example, we can choose whom to marry, how many children to have, what religion to follow, where to live, how to spend our leisure time, and what doctors to solicit for our medical needs. This concept of privacy protects us from undue interference with our lives by governmental agencies or others in general. We all need to respect each other's privacy (Behnke, Perlin, & Bernstein, 2003).

Confidentiality is related to privacy. For our purposes here, I will discuss the notion of confidentiality as it relates to doctor-patient relationships. When a person visits a mental health professional such as a psychologist or psychiatrist, he or she must have assurance that whatever is being communicated to these doctors will not be disclosed to anybody, or to any entity. While assurance of confidentiality is always important when one seeks medical consultation, it is especially significant in the mental health arena. When patients interact with mental health providers they typically reveal the most intimate aspects of their personal life, and even sensitive features of other people's life with whom they may have come in contact. Exceptions to confidentiality do exist. There are times when the law authorizes a breach of confidentiality in order to assure certain important social

240

interests. Examples of these are treatment emergencies, public safety, peer and administrative review, the needs of the legal system, facilitation of research, and mandatory reporting statutes (Behnke, Perlin, & Bernstein, 2003). I will now briefly elaborate on these exceptions. When treatment emergencies arise, health related information is urgently needed in order to properly and safely treat a patient. For example, prior to filling out a new prescription, an emergency room physician may need to know what kind of medication the patient has been taking, in order to avoid dangerous medication interactions. In such situations there is no time to sort out the legalities linked to confidentiality issues.

The law allows for safety measures to be taken, when a mentally ill patient intends to harm a third party. For example, if in the course of psychotherapy a patient states that she will stab her husband with a knife upon her arrival home, the treating psychologist, psychiatrist or any other mental health professional has the freedom to notify the husband or the police of the patient's intentions. The law allows certain supervising agencies to review the treatments patients receive in clinics, hospitals and other mental health related institutions. The purpose of this review is to assure that patients get quality care from mental health professionals. This administrative process involves examination of records and discussions with doctors and other providers of mental health services about the care patients receive.

Medical research is needed to advance our knowledge related to the etiology, diagnosis and treatment of mental diseases. In order to facilitate their work, researches need to have access to patients, and to their medical and treatment histories. While the law does not require anyone to participate in research studies, patients may elect to participate. Should patients choose to participate, their identities will not be disclosed. Furthermore, researchers are required to inform patients about the nature and purpose of the study, the duration of the study, and any risks involved. Patients have the right to withdraw from a study at any time.

The purpose of mandatory reporting statutes is to provide protection for particularly vulnerable individuals, such as children, severely retarded individuals, elderly sick persons, and patients with severe mental disorders. When harm, neglect or abuse is detected, information about these patients must be promptly reported to those agencies responsible for their protection.

It is important to note that competent patients always have the right to request that information about their condition and treatment be released to *specifically named* individuals or agencies. When such a request is made it is necessary for the named recipient of confidential information to demonstrate a *need* for such information. The *consent* of the patient related to such disclosures must be *received* by the person or entity needing the information. Furthermore, the treating mental health professional must reasonably determine that sharing of confidential information will not harm the client. The *Health Insurance Portability and Accountability Act of 1996 (HIPAA)* was enacted by the United States Congress in part to protect the privacy and security of protected health information. Patients are advised to become familiar with the details of this act. Information may be obtained from the United States Department of Health and Human Services (HHS.gov).

Testimonial privilege is also related to the concepts of privacy and autonomy. Specifically, patients have the right to keep confidential information related to their psychiatric condition from being disclosed in a legal proceeding. No information discussed with a mental health professional may be disclosed without the patient's explicit permission. This means that a treating professional may not release a patient's records, nor may he testify about matters related to his patient in a court of law (Behnke, Perlin, & Bernstein, 2003).

There are exceptions to testimonial privilege. Four examples follow: 1. When a psychiatrist or psychologist believes that an outpatient is in need of hospitalization but the patient disagrees, the treating doctor may be required to testify in court about the patient's condition and the need for hospitalization. 2. There are legal cases where an individual's mental health needs to be established. Depending on his mental status a person may or may not be competent to be tried in a court of law. Hence before a trial can proceed the court can order that the person be examined by a qualified mental health professional. 3. Similarly, in a criminal case the court may order that a defendant be given a mental status examination in order to determine criminal responsibility for a committed act of crime. 4. In certain civil cases individuals waive testimonial privilege. These are cases where emotional damages are claimed. Here again a mental health evaluation must be performed (Behnke, Perlin, & Bernstein, 2003).

Competent adults and children regardless of whether they are inpatients or outpatients have the right to *informed consent* to treatment. This simply means that the treating professional must apprise them of the nature of the evaluation and treatment they are going to get. The potential risks and benefits of the evaluation and treatment must be discussed. Alternatives to the intervention, including risks and benefits also need to be explained. The anticipated length of treatment may warrant discussion as well. Voluntary patients have the right to refuse treatment. Should they refuse certain types of treatment, court ordered patients have the right to a *judicial review* of their treatment plan.

When a patient feels that her rights have been violated, or that she has suffered damages in the course of treatment, she has the right to bring a lawsuit against the treating mental health professional or against a mental health facility. The statute of limitations in such cases should be discussed with an attorney. In general legal action against physicians must be initiated within two and one half years following the last date of treatment. In the case of psychologists the statute of limitations is three years (Behnke, Perlin, & Bernstein, 2003). Given the frequently elusive and intangible nature of psychiatric treatment, claimed damages should be carefully documented and dated. Only specialized and experienced attorneys should be consulted when contemplating this type of legal action.

SECTION 8.3:
CIVIL COMMITMENT

The following topics are discussed in this section:
The responsibility of the state to its citizens with regard to
mental illness
The definition of "dangerousness" in the context of mental
illness
The legal rights of patients in a psychiatric hospital
The function of the Mental Hygiene Legal Service
Patients' rights regarding refusal to take psychotropic
medications
The right to refuse electroconvulsive treatment (ECT)
The rights of children in a psychiatric hospital
Laws related to the restraint and seclusion of psychiatri-
cally hospitalized patients

As citizens living in a democratic society, we treasure our personal liberties. We have laws, which guarantee our freedom. Our government has the obligation to protect us from harm, and to assure our safety. But what happens when a person becomes mentally ill, and as a consequence of her illness she is unable to take care of her daily needs, and is unable to protect herself? What happens if she becomes suicidal or starts to physically threaten others? What is the responsibility of the government in such cases? Basically in such instances the government must protect and facilitate the provision of psychiatric care for the sick person. Concurrently, the government must also protect the public from the dangerous behaviors of mentally ill individuals.

There are times when mentally sick persons require hospitalization, but they refuse to be hospitalized. Such refusal may simply be an indication that the patient has very impaired judgment, and has no understanding of the services a hospital can provide. Some patients, on the other hand, may be adverse to the idea of confinement and loss of personal freedom. In such situations the state can resort to two sorts of endowed powers in order to carry out its duty. The first type of power is called *parens patriae*. This doctrine dates back to Roman law. England acquired this law around the eleventh century. This power authorizes the state to act like a parent, and to care for citizens who are unable to care for themselves (Weiner & Hess, 2006).

The second type of power is called *police power*. This power authorizes the state to detain people who are dangerous to themselves or to others. In the present time civil commitment to a psychiatric hospital involves the establishment of *dangerousness*. The presence of mental illness by itself is not considered sufficient cause for *involuntary hospitalization*. It is important, however to understand the broad interpretation of dangerousness. A patient who is suicidal or homicidal is certainly dangerous. But when a patent's mental condition is so deteriorated that he is unable to perform essential daily activities such as buying food, taking needed medication, getting dressed, or living in a sheltered environment, then too a patient is considered to be dangerous, and may require hospitalization. It is important to note that civilly committed patients have the right to an attorney. They also have the right to automatic periodic court review of their psychiatric condition to determine the need for continued involuntary hospitalization. Initial court ordered retentions for involuntary hospitalization may be up to a period of six months. When needed, the retention order may be extended for an additional twelve-month period, and then again extended for additional twenty-four month periods (Behnke, Perlin, & Bernstein, 2003).

The Mental Hygiene Legal Service (MHLS) provides legal advice to persons receiving inpatient psychiatric care. This is a free service provided by the New York State court system. When hospitalized patients do not have private lawyers, the attorneys of the MHLS will advise patients of their rights related to the treatment they are receiving. These attorneys have unqualified access to all patient records and to hospital employees who provide psychiatric treatment. In court hearings where patients complain about their treatment or challenge their involuntary hospital status, lawyers of the MHLS can represent them (Behnke, Perlin, & Bernstein, 2003).

It is important to be familiar with the various types of admission to a psychiatric hospital. Besides involuntary hospitalization discussed above, there are several others. *Informal admission* requires no formal written application. An informal patient is free to leave the hospital at any time during ordinary business hours. Should an informal patient decide to stay in the hospital, he may be converted to any other suitable legal status. A *voluntary admission* to a psychiatric hospital involves a written request on the part of the patient for hospitalization. The law requires of them to understand that they are making an application for admission to a psychiatric facility. They also need to understand the meaning of voluntary status, the requirements for discharge from the hospital, and the possibility for conversion to involuntary status. Voluntary patients do not enjoy the automatic periodic judicial review offered to involuntary patients. When a voluntary patient wishes to leave the hospital, she must submit a *72-hour letter*. The 72-hour letter is basically a written demand by a patient for immediate release. In essence this letter gives the director of the hospital 72 hours to either discharge the patient, or submit an application to the court for an order of retention. When such an application is made, it must be supported by the certificates of two examining physicians. The patient must remain in the hospital until the date of the retention hearing. The court may either approve or reject the application for retention.

An *emergency admission* is appropriate when a patient committed a recent dangerous act, or exhibited dangerous behavior towards herself or others. Hostile, threatening verbal behavior and destruction of property may constitute dangerous conduct. Inability to carry out activities of daily living, as described above may also necessitate emergency admission. Emergency admissions usually entail involuntary legal status. These patients may be retained up to fifteen days for observation and psychiatric care. If further retention is needed, a court order must be procured. There may come a time when an individual feels the need to have another person involuntarily hospitalized. In order for this to happen, the person earmarked for admission must be examined by two physicians in order to determine the need for inpatient care.

Any person who shares residence with a mentally ill person may apply for a *2-P.C. admission*. Relatives, or a court appointed guardian of a mentally ill patient may also apply. Such applications must not be frivolous! The reasons for the application must be clearly stated and must be truthful! Detailed facts are needed enumerating the reasons that one believes that another person is mentally ill and needs treatment. Providing false information is tantamount to a criminal act, which is punishable by law! A patient may remain in a hospital on a 2-P.C. admission status for a period of sixty days. At any time during this sixty-day period a court hearing may be requested. The patient, his attorney, the MHLS, any friend or relative of the patient, or the person who originally initiated the involuntary hospitalization process may make such a request. The request must be submitted in writing to the director of the hospital. If in the opinion of the treatment team the patient needs further treatment, the director of the hospital may petition the court for an order of retention (Behnke, Perlin, & Bernstein, 2003).

In our democratic type of government the preservation of basic civil rights is held in great esteem. These rights are extended to mentally ill persons as well. Suppose a patient disagrees with the hospital's decision to provide involuntary treatment; what legal options does this patient have? The law provides the right for patients to challenge their involuntary status. A court hearing may be scheduled for this purpose. The patient is then represented by either a private attorney or the MHLS. The patient is required to provide reasons for their objections to hospitalization; she must convince the court that her state of mind and behavior poses no danger to herself or to others. The hospital must bring evidence to the contrary. After listening to both parties the judge makes the decision. What actions can a patient take if he is dissatisfied with the judge's decision? Here again the law protects the rights of patients! A patient has the option to challenge a judge's decision and may request a new trial by a jury. Alternatively, the patient may waive the jury, and seek a new hearing before a different judge. At this new hearing fresh evidence related to the patient's condition must be presented to the court by both parties.

Patients also have the freedom to forego a rehearing, and appeal the initial judge's decision to an appellate court. Likewise, a rehearing may also be appealed (Behnke, Perlin, & Bernstein, 2003).

During the course of their hospitalization patients have clearly defined *rights*! Primarily they are entitled to a clean, safe environment and freedom from abuse by staff. They must be treated in a humane and respectful manner. They must be offered nutritious meals and appropriate clothing. They must be given privacy in bathing and in toilet areas. They must be allowed to practice their religion. They must be allowed privacy during visiting hours, and be allowed to send and receive mail, and to use the telephone to communicate with people outside the hospital. Hospitalized patients have the right to ask for another opinion from a private physician about their treatment. They have the right to read their medical records with their treating doctor unless he believes that doing so could harm the patient. Patients have the right to refuse participation in research projects without suffering any negative consequences arising from their refusal. Patients also have the right to participate in the development of their individualized treatment plan. A periodic (at least yearly) evaluation of patients and a review of their treatment plan is mandated. In addition to the psychiatric care they are receiving, they are also entitled to appropriate medical and dental care. Upon admission to the hospital, staff must familiarize patients with these rights. A list of these rights must be posted in each ward of the hospital (Behnke, Perlin, & Bernstein, 2003).

Throughout their psychiatric hospitalization patients have a number of *responsibilities*. They, and in many cases, their significant others need to provide accurate information about matters related to their physical and mental health. Perceived risks in their care must be reported as well. Patients need to notify members of their treatment team if they do not understand their diagnosis, any details of their treatment plan, or prognosis. They need to notify their treatment team if they do not wish to see certain visitors, or to receive telephone calls. They need to respect the privacy and safety of other patients. They are expected to abide by the smoking policy of the facility.

They are expected to follow their prescribed plan of treatment and care. Patients need to voice any dissatisfaction regarding their care or violation of their rights. They are responsible to meet their financial obligations to the hospital.

We know that mental illness may be caused by psychological, social, or biological factors, or by the interaction of these three. We use treatment modalities to address all three factors. When there is good reason to believe that significant biological causes underlie a person's mental disorder, it is customary to offer *medication* to a patient. However some patients do not like the idea of ingesting drugs which control their brain function. Others may have a hard time tolerating the side effects of medication.

Do hospitalized patients have the *right to refuse* antipsychotic or any other psychoactive medication? To answer this question we need to consider the legal status of the patient. Informal and voluntary patients have the right to refuse pharmacological treatment, as well as any other treatment. The only exception to this rule is an emergency situation where the administration of medication becomes necessary in order to prevent physical harm to self or others. Patients who are on an involuntary status also have the right to refuse medication! Unless there is an emergency situation, an involuntary patient may not be medicated against his will. When a treating psychiatrist in a hospital feels that a patient needs medication in order to optimally treat his mental illness, and the patient refuses to comply, the hospital then must request a court hearing. At that hearing the hospital must prove that the patient is not competent to determine her own treatment. The hospital must also explain to the court the expected benefits and risks that will result from taking medication. The type and dosage of the proposed medication must be disclosed at the hearing. Any alternatives to medicating the patient must also be stated. The court will either approve, disapprove, or modify the proposed treatment. Such court orders are time limited, and must be reviewed periodically (Behnke, Perlin, & Bernstein, 2003).

There are times when neither psychotherapy nor medications are effective in treating a patient. *Electroconvulsive treatment (ECT)* may be another option. Voluntary and informal patients may refuse this type of treatment. Involuntary patients may also refuse. If the hospital feels that ECT is absolutely the right choice of treatment, then a court hearing must be scheduled. At the hearing the hospital must provide evidence that the patient is incompetent to determine his own treatment. Reasons must also be given for choosing ECT as a treatment modality, as opposed to less invasive methods. Here again the judge will either accept, reject, or modify the recommended treatment. Court orders for ECT are time limited, and must be reviewed periodically. It is important to know that the law does not allow electroconvulsive treatment on an emergency basis (Behnke, Perlin, & Bernstein, 2003).

Involuntary hospitalization also applies to *children*. When children are hospitalized against their will, the law provides them with the exact same protection as adults get. Although treatment decisions are reserved for parents, regardless of age, a child may demand a court hearing. An attorney will represent him, and a judge will rule on his case. If he is displeased with the judge's decision, the child may ask for a jury to review his case. He may also ask for a different judge to hear his case. Parental consent or a court order is needed before any psychotropic medication is administered to children. When a child (under the age of eighteen) refuses to take medication, his condition and treatment plan will be reviewed administratively in the hospital. In such cases a court appearance is not required. Sixteen and seventeen year old individuals may admit themselves to a psychiatric hospital on a voluntary basis with the consent of the hospital director. Children under the age of sixteen need their parents or guardians to apply for admission on their behalf. A minor voluntary patient has the right to request release from the hospital with a 72-hour letter. A parent, relative or the MHLS may also ask for the discharge of the child (Behnke, Perlin, & Bernstein, 2003).

During the course of their hospitalization patients may become *physically dangerous* to themselves or to others. They may become violent, or attempt suicidal acts. As a preventive measure patients may be restrained or secluded. A camisole or restraining sheet may be used when restraint is indicated for a patient. These devices prevent free physical movement. Patients may not be restrained for more than two hours on a continuous basis. Periodic supervision by staff must be provided. When a patient in restraint is asleep, he must be kept under constant supervision (eye contact by a staff member). For a sleeping patient the two-hour limit does not apply. Secluded patients are placed in a room alone with closed door. The door cannot be opened from the inside. Periodic supervision by staff must be in place. Patients may not be secluded for more than three hours on a continuous basis, unless they are asleep. Ward staff must visit sleeping patients every hour both day and night. Restraint and seclusion may only be used if less restrictive methods have not worked to prevent injury. A physician must document the precise reasons for writing an order of restraint or seclusion. These restrictive ways may never be used as a means of behavior modification or punishment. Persons with the sole diagnosis of mental retardation may not be secluded. If they also have a secondary diagnosis of mental illness, then seclusion may be used if less restrictive methods prove to be insufficient to prevent harm (Behnke, Perlin, & Bernstein, 2003).

SECTION 8.4:
ASSISTED OUTPATIENT TREATMENT

The following topics are discussed in this section:
The definition of assisted outpatient treatment
Who benefits from assisted outpatient treatment
The legal steps necessary to receive assisted outpatient
treatment
The consequence of non-compliance with assisted outpatient treatment

In many cases mentally sick patients do not comply with recommended outpatient treatment. Consequently they may become self-destructive, violent, and may pose a danger to themselves or others. *Assisted outpatient treatment (AOT)* or *outpatient commitment* requires patients to observe their treatment plan. This may involve taking medications, receiving psychotherapy, living in a supervised setting, or attending a day mental health program. Patients with a diagnosis of alcohol or substance abuse may be required to submit to blood or urine test monitoring. Patients with histories of repeated inpatient hospitalizations who have not adhered to outpatient treatment regimes often benefit from AOT. Many patients who receive court ordered outpatient treatment cannot manage their daily activities for safe living in the community. In New York State assisted outpatient treatment is court ordered, and must be the least restrictive effective treatment deemed necessary for the patient's psychiatric condition. Non-compliance with this court order alone cannot be a reason for involuntary hospitalization. Likewise, non-compliance with AOT is not punishable by law (Behnke, Perlin, & Bernstein, 2003).

Any adult person (at least 18 years of age) may go to court and ask that a particular individual with whom they reside be ordered to receive assisted outpatient treatment. Close relatives (parents, children, siblings, spouses) of the designated subject may also file petitions with the court. Probation and parole officers enjoy the same right vis-à-vis those they supervise. All applications for AOT must be supported by convincing evidence from the applicant that a particular person needs this type of service. A physician's evaluation and court testimony are needed as well. The court may deny or grant petitions. Initial court orders may not exceed a duration of six months. Additional orders have a limit of one year. All AOT patients must have an individualized treatment plan. Patients have the right to participate in the development of their treatment plans. Case managers encourage and supervise patients to abide by their plan of treatment. They also monitor patients' clinical progress, and the need for modifications in the treatment plan. Significant proposed changes in patient care require a court order. If as a result of non-compliance with AOT, or otherwise, a patient's mental condition deteriorates to such a degree that outpatient treatment is no longer effective, inpatient hospitalization may be recommended, and legally enforced if needed (Behnke, Perlin, & Bernstein, 2003).

SECTION 8.5:
CRIMINAL LAW

The following topics are discussed in this section:
The legal management of defendants who are incompetent
to stand trial
The meaning and legal management of the insanity defense

There are two important considerations related to criminal behavior that are worthy of exploration. The first item has to do with *competence to stand trial and competence to plead guilty (adjudicative competence)*. In order for a person to be fit to stand trial he must understand the nature of the judicial proceedings. He needs to comprehend the role of the prosecutor, the defense attorney, the jury, and the judge. He must be able to rationally discuss his case with his lawyer (Greene et al., 2007). He also must understand the accusations he is facing. Furthermore a defendant must be able to comprehend the consequences of pleading guilty, and must be able to rationally decide to go to trial or not to do so.

When a defendant's competence becomes an issue, the court will order a psychiatric examination by two qualified professionals, who can be psychiatrists or psychologists. The court will then decide on the defendant's competence to stand trial based on these clinical evaluations. Incompetent defendants with *misdemeanor* charges will enjoy the necessary dismissal of their charges. They will then be required to undergo a 72-hour observation period by mental health professionals employed by the State Office of Mental Health (OMH), or the State Office of Mental Retardation and Developmental Disabilities (OMRDD). If needed, they will receive treatment in either an inpatient state facility or on an outpatient basis. Incompetent defendants with *felony* charges will receive a court order of commitment to an OMH specialized forensic hospital or to an OMRDD facility. This order is valid up to six months. When more time is required, a 12-month order of retention will follow suit. Further retention orders are valid for two-year periods. Once a defendant is "restored to competency" and is fit to stand trial, he will be required to face the charges against him in court. "When a person remains incompetent for two-thirds of the maximum term to which he could have been sentenced for the highest crime charged against him, the charges are dismissed" (Behnke, Perlin, & Bernstein, 2003).

The second item related to criminal behavior has to do with *criminal responsibility*. In New York State the law states that a person should not be held responsible for his criminal conduct if at the time of the criminal act, as a result of mental illness, he "lacked substantial capacity to know or appreciate the nature and consequences of his conduct, or that his conduct was wrong." (Behnke, Perlin, & Bernstein, 2003). An example may be a person who, in response to a command hallucination, physically attacks another individual. As another example, a patient with bipolar disorder in a manic episode may decide to steal a bicycle in an attempt to ride it cross country from New York to California in two days. A psychiatric evaluation is a necessary component to the substantiation of an insanity defense. (Weiner & Hess, 2006). If the court finds a person not responsible for a criminal offense, then the court will commit the person to the OMH or to the OMRDD for treatment. Individuals whose mental illness poses a danger to themselves or others will be committed to a secure psychiatric facility. The court will order these defendants to strictly comply with their plan of treatment (Behnke, Perlin, & Bernstein, 2003).

EPILOGUE

Upon reviewing the eight chapters of this manuscript I feel that I have accomplished my initial intention. I have addressed the topics which have both an educational and practical value to those who are interested in basic psychological phenomena relevant to daily life, as well as to the span of life. Areas related to development, parenting, and relationships have been explored in some detail. The effects of stress, the nature of common mental illnesses, the description of mental health providers, diagnostic techniques, and treatment modalities have also been discussed. Finally, I also touched upon issues related to the intersection of mental illness and the law.

The brain is the most complex and least understood organ in the body. The products of the brain—mental processes and observable behaviors—are also very difficult to fully understand. Our psychological processes are a function of evolution, genetics, physiological variables, the environment in which we live, and the opportunities for learning offered to us. There are still many topics related to the human psyche that could be opened for discussion in this book. Now that much of the essentials have been covered, it will be easier for me to add to this foundation in future editions.

While this book serves as a valuable guide to the prevention and solution of a variety of problems, let us not forget that common sense is often the answer to difficulties we encounter in daily life. Looking back and learning from our experiences, and reflecting upon the teachings of our parents and grandparents can give clues to the solution of many of our dilemmas. Undeniably we live in a technologically and scientifically more advanced world than our mothers, and fathers did. But the basic nature of human beings has not changed. Essential psychological tools for success and proper adjustment have remained the same over the passage of time.

Let us be active thinkers rather than robotic creatures! Let us keep self-exploration alive! Let us not lose important perspectives in life! Let us learn from the lives of our ancestors; let us learn from our mistakes and successes, and from the mistakes and successes of others! Answers to existential and philosophical questions such as, "Who am I?", or "What is the meaning and purpose of my life?", or "What is the meaning of 'meaning'?" are difficult to find. But deep thinking, contemplation, and reasoning stimulate and feed our intellect and spirit! In many ways we all are the sculptors of our lives and the lives of those with whom we interact. We mutually influence those with whom we share our life space. We are all builders of the social structure in which we live. We humans are interdependent and rely on one another as we strive to attain our daily needs. We must be flexible, open-minded, and cooperate with one another to assure our well-being, to promote social, scientific and technological progress, and to maintain a harmonious balance between what we take and what we contribute as members of our social network on this earth.

APPENDIX I

CHILD ABUSE RELATED RESOURCES RECOMMENDED BY THE AMERICAN PSYCHOLOGICAL ASSOCIATION:

American Professional Society on the Abuse of Children
407 South Dearborn, Suite 1300
Chicago, IL 60605
(312-554-0166
www.apsac.org

National Center for Missing and Exploited Children
Charles B. Wang International Children's Building
699 Prince Street
Alexandria, VA 22314-3175
24-hour hotline: 1-800-THE-LOST
www.missingkids.com

Child Help USA
15757 North 78th Street
Scottsdale, AZ 85260
1-800-4-A-CHILD
www.childhelpusa.org

National Clearinghouse on Child Abuse and Neglect Information, U.S. Department of Health and Human Services
P.O.Box 1182
Washington, DC 20013
1-800-FYI-3366
www.calib.com/nccanch

Prevent Child Abuse America
332 S. Michigan Avenue, Suite 1600
Chicago, IL 60604-4357
1-800-CHILDREN
www.preventchildabuse.org

APPENDIX II

SUGGESTIONS ON HOW TO IDENTIFY HIGH QUALITY AND APPROPRIATE DAY CARE CENTERS

It is important to ask providers of service detailed questions without feeling embarrassed or inhibited. Caregivers and center administrators who are proud of their services will freely answer all questions, and give you an introductory tour of their facility. Many centers will provide brochures with exact description of their services and qualifications of their staff.

The following agenda items should be considered prior to deciding on a day care facility:

- Licensure: What licensing agency issued the operating license? What were the licensure requirements?

- What is the census of the center (how many infants are actively enrolled)? How many caregivers are employed? One caregiver for every four infants is optimal. The ratio may be higher for older children.

- What kind of education and training did caregivers receive? Do they speak correct and fluent English? Did they have training in the physical and behavioral needs of infants and children? Did the center administration check employees' references and credentials? Are the caregivers proactive and interactive? Do they attempt to engage children in educational and creative activities? Are they motivated and enjoy their work? Qualified day-care workers are often difficult to find, because they are often underpaid, or "off the books" illegal non-English speaking immigrants.

- Physical environmental concerns are also very important. Is the facility safe and secure? Are children protected from strangers walking in unnoticed? Is there a fire alarm system? When was it last inspected? Is there an unobstructed emergency exit? Is the facility "child-proof"? Are there any hazardous substances, sharp objects, or unprotected electrical outlets? Is the furniture in good condition? Are games, toys and art supplies safely stored when not in use? Is the environment clean and well illuminated? What kind of meals and snacks are served? Are they healthy and appetizing? For younger infants, what formulas are used?

- What kind of infants and children attend this center? Are there any exclusion criteria for admission?

- Are there sufficient toys, books, art and craft materials, and board games? Is the environment stimulating and pleasant to the senses?

- Is there space for physical activities, such as swinging, cycling, sliding? Is proper supervision provided during physical play activities?

- Are the center's operating hours convenient for working parents? Is the center located relatively close to home?

- Are parents allowed to visit unannounced? Is it possible to meet with the caregivers who will be assigned to your infant? It is advised to insist on these meetings.

- These and any other questions should be asked freely and without feelings of intrusion.

APPENDIX III

THEORIES OF PERSONALITY DEVELOPMENT

The following is a summary of some of the major personality theories used today by clinicians and behavioral scientists to describe and explain the characteristics that make children and adults unique as individuals:

1. *Psychoanalytic Theory*: This was the first major theory of personality, proposed by Sigmund Freud over 110 years ago. He theorized that the mind consists of three levels of consciousness: the conscious, the preconscious, and the unconscious. He held that personality and behavior are shaped by unconscious forces and conflicts. He claimed that the interaction of the *id, ego* and *superego* determines the quality of our behavior and coping abilities in life. The id is a psychic structure present at birth, and contains our basic drives for survival, and instinctual impulses. The function of the ego is to balance the instinctual demands of the id with social realities and expectations. The ego forms during the first year of life. The superego first appears between ages three and five. Its function is to ensure moral and conscientious behavior. According to Freud, children go through five *psychosexual* stages of development: The *oral,* anal, *phallic, latency,* and *genital* stages. These stages are called "psychosexual" in nature, because they are characterized by changes in how the child derives pleasure from erogenous (sexually sensitive) parts of the body. Proper and relatively conflict-free passage through these stages are necessary for optimal psychological adjustment later in life. Unresolved conflicts, which arise from receiving insufficient or excessive gratification, may lead to adjustment problems or mental illness later in life. (Nevid, 2013).

2. *Theory of Ego Psychology*: Ego theorists such as Erik Erikson, emphasize the strengths and abilities of the ego, as well as societal forces, which shape personality. The construct of "identity" is considered a vital need of every human being. Identity gives us a sense of uniqueness and inner wholeness. It also allows us to experience life in a consistent fashion with a logical chronological continuity from the past through the present and into the future. Individuals with a well crystallized identity will feel a sense of social recognition, belonging and support. Erikson stated that personality development is a life-long process, and can be conceptualized in eight stages from infancy to old age. Every stage involves a "crisis" (specific problem), which is created by the child's increasing physical maturity, and the accompanying parental and societal expectations and demands. The successful compliance with these novel expectations depends on continued ego functioning, which is necessary for a healthy personality development (Ewen, 2003).

3. *Trait Theory*: Trait theorists such as Gordon W. Allport believe that personality can best be understood in terms of relatively stable and enduring characteristics or dispositions, called *traits*. These traits reside within the individual. Responsibility and friendliness are examples of traits, but there are many others, which define our unique personalities and styles of behavior (Ewen, 2003).

4. *Humanistic Theory*: Carl Rogers and Abraham Maslow underscore the importance of our inborn potentials to flourish in a natural and uninterrupted manner. This is called *self-actualization*. Excessive parental and societal pressures may block this developmental flow, and may result in our inability to set independent goals. This may lead to unhappiness and even mental illness. Nonjudgmental, positive, and minimally critical attitudes of parents toward their children are essential for a healthy personality development. Rather than imposing their own values and wishes, parents need to facilitate and guide their children toward self-knowledge, and allow them to develop their individual skills and goals (Ewen, 2003).

APPENDIX IV

DISEASES THAT CHILDHOOD VACCINES PREVENT

Diphtheria (4 doses)
Haemophilus influenzae, type b (3-4 doses)
Hepatitis A (2 doses)
Hepatitis B (3 doses)
Influenza (2-3 doses)
Measles (1 dose)
Meningococcal
Mumps (1 dose)
Pertussis (4 doses)
Pneumococcal (4 doses)
Polio (3 doses)
Rotavirus (3 doses)
Rubella (1 dose)
Tetanus (4 doses)
Varicella (1 dose)

General immunization questions can be answered in both English and Spanish by the Centers for Disease Control at 1-800-232-4636. (Rathus, 2008)

**It is important to consult your pediatrician
regarding the above information.**

APPENDIX V

MINIMIZING THE RISK OF LEAD POISONING

Children can ingest lead by putting objects covered with led dust in their mouths, or by eating paint chips, or breathing in lead dust. In order to prevent lead poisoning, it is important to know where lead is found. House paint is a major source of lead. In 1978 the federal government banned the use of lead-based paint. Many homes built prior to the institution of this ban may have used lead containing paint. Where else can lead be found? The following is a partial list of lead containing surfaces, materials, and objects:

- Soil surrounding a dwelling
- Household dust
- Drinking water
- Household plumbing
- Old furniture and toy paint
- Lead-glazed pottery or porcelain
- Air near industrial sites

Some suggestions for precautions and prevention:

- Use only cold water for drinking or cooking. Run water for about twenty seconds before drinking it.
- Have your water tested by the health department.
- Do not use lead-glazed food containers.
- Peeling lead-based paint needs immediate repair.
- Arrange for a paint inspection of your home
- Ask your pediatrician to have your child tested for lead levels in the body.

For more information contact the National Lead Information Center.
Phone: 1-800-424-5323
E-mail: http://www.epa.gov/lead/pubs/nlic.htm
(Rathus, 2008)

APPENDIX VI

SUGGESTIONS FOR GUIDING AND CONTROLLING YOUNG CHILDREN'S BEHAVIOR

- Explain the rules and regulations patiently, using language that children can understand; be concrete, and use examples if needed.

- Rules, regulations, and expectations should be reasonable and age appropriate.

- When talking to your child, sit down and look into his/her eyes.

- Repeat and remind your child important expectations as often as needed, preferably in the beginning of each day.

- Recognize and reward (a nice word, a hug, or an added privilege) good behavior.

- When using punishment such as "time out", explain the reason(s) for it twice: first, when punishment begins, and again when it ends, making sure that the child understands it.

- Avoid excessive punishment, and punishment which is out of proportion with the mischief or violation.

- When promising rewards or punishments, carry them out in a timely manner.

- Rewards and punishments should be consistent and immediate. Good behavior should be closely and consistently followed by reward. Similarly, wrongdoings should be closely and consistently followed by punishment.

- Ignore negative or annoying behaviors such as nagging, whining or tantrums. Remember that an angry response may be reinforcing. Paying no attention consistently may extinguish the unwanted behavior.

- Avoid reprimanding your child when you are tired, not feeling good, stressed, pressed for time, or angry.

- Do not fight with your spouse or use abusive language in the presence of your child. Remember that children will imitate what they see.

- Avoid excessive "lecturing", shaming and guilt induction.

- Dangerous and breakable items should be out of reach.

- Avoid making comparisons, such as "Look how nicely your brother is playing; why can't you be like him?"

- Find alternatives for unwanted behaviors. Rather than just saying "Stop watching television!" propose an alternative activity, such as a game board, or riding a bicycle.

APPENDIX VII

WEIGHT MANAGEMENT SUGGESTIONS
FOR OVERWEIGHT CHILDREN

According to the literature on weight management, the following methods are useful in the prevention of weight gain, and in weight reduction efforts:

- Educate children about the essentials of proper nutrition (see below), and the meaning of terms such as calories, protein, vitamins, minerals, fibers, and food groups.

- Allow children to eat when they are hungry, rather than at specific times during the day. For example, do not insist that they should eat dinner because "now is dinner time".

- High-calorie foods must be avoided. Low-calorie foods must be substituted. If in doubt, consult a nutritionist for appropriate meal planning and preparation.

- Serve moderate size portions, and do not offer second helpings.

- Allow children to stop eating when they feel full, even if there is still food left on their plate. A little "waste" is preferable to overeating.

- Prepare low-calorie snacks to eat throughout the day, to prevent binge eating.

- Try to avoid cooking, eating or displaying fattening foods when children are at home, especially when they are hungry. The sight and aroma of foods may be tempting.

- Keep children busy with a variety of activities. When the mind is occupied, fantasizing about food is minimized.

- Do not take children to stores or supermarkets for food shopping.

- Ask relatives and friends to refrain from offering fattening treats.

- Firmly discourage snacking while watching television shows, or while sitting in front of a computer.

- Habitually involve children in physical play or exercise activities, such as running, dancing, swimming or bicycle riding.

- Devise a simple behavior modification program aimed at rewarding proper eating behaviors and physical activities. Be consistent in recognizing and reinforcing children's efforts in the desired direction.

- Accidental "slips" should be forgiven and discussed, rather than punished or admonished.

- Discuss briefly the importance of weight management and physical fitness frequently, preferably daily in the morning, until proper dietary habits are acquired. Avoid "preaching", excessive "warnings", and "comparing" a child's progress in weight loss to that of other children.

- As a parent, be a positive model to your children. Follow a sensible diet and healthy lifestyle. If needed, lose weight together with your child. This will result in added and sustained motivation.

Essentials of proper nutrition:

1. Green vegetables and fruit may be consumed in large quantities (suitable for snacks throughout the day)
2. Low or non-fat milk products.
3. Roasted or baked poultry with skin removed.
4. Low-fat baked or broiled fish.
5. Pasta and beans (in moderate amounts).
6. Whole grain cereals and nuts (in moderate amounts).
7. Low-fat pork and beef (rarely in small amounts)
8. Low-fat salad dressing and olive oil (in small amounts)
9. Avoid all fried foods, butter, margarine, mayonnaise, and high sugar and carbohydrate desert items such as cakes and ice cream.
10. Avoid sweet beverages and alcohol.
11. Drink water regularly.

It is important to consult your pediatrician and dietitian regarding the above information!

APPENDIX VIII

COMMONLY USED INTELLIGENCE TESTS

Stanford-Binet Intelligence Scale-V: The fifth and most recent revision of this test took place in 2003. The test is suitable for individuals from age 2 to age 85 and even older. The test measures both verbal and non-verbal abilities. The combined score of the five verbal subtests yields a Verbal IQ. The combined score of the five nonverbal subtests yields a Nonverbal IQ. Scores on all ten subtests yield a Full Scale IQ. The test measures both verbal and nonverbal reasoning, knowledge, quantitative reasoning, visual-spatial processing, and working memory. The total administration time for the test is one hour.

Wechsler Intelligence Tests: The Wechsler Adult Intelligence Scale (WAIS-IV) is suitable for individuals aged 16 to 89. The test is comprised of seven verbal and seven performance (nonverbal) subtests. Verbal, performance, and full scale IQs can be calculated. The test measures four major cognitive abilities (indexes); these are, verbal reasoning and comprehension, working memory, processing speed, and perceptual organization (ability to solve nonverbal information). It takes approximately one and one-half hours to complete this test. The Wechsler Intelligence Scale for Children (WISC) was designed for children between the ages of 6 and 16 years 11 months. WISC-IV, the latest update of this instrument was introduced in 2003. The test consists of ten core subtests and five optional subtests, and measures the same major cognitive abilities (indexes) as the WAIS. The WISC-IV yields four index scores and a full scale IQ. It takes approximately one and one-half hours to complete this test. The Wechsler Preschool and Primary Scale of Intelligence (WPPSI-III) was published in 2002. It was designed to be administered to children between the ages of 2 years and 6 months and 7 years and 3 months. The test consists of fifteen subtests, measuring both verbal and nonverbal skills. The test yields verbal, performance and full scale IQs. The test can be completed between 30 and 60 minutes, depending on the age of the child (younger children usually require less time) (Aiken & Groth-Marnat, 2006).

Less frequently used intelligence tests include the following:

- Detroit Test of Learning Aptitude
- Kaufman's Intelligence Tests
- Woodcock-Johnson III Tests of Cognitive Abilities

APPENDIX IX

PROGRAMS AND SUPPORT FOR PREGNANT TEENAGERS

The following agencies provide legal, medical, psychological, or social services for pregnant teenagers:

- NATIONAL CENTER FOR YOUTH LAW
  405 14TH Street
  Oakland, CA 94612
  Phone: 510-835-8098

- THE U.S. DEPARTMENT OF HEALTH AND HUMAN SERVICES
  200 Independence Avenue, S.W.
  Washington, D.C. 20201
  Phone: 1-877-696-6775

PROGRAMS FOR THE PREVENTION OF TEENAGE PREGNANCY

The following agencies provide information, preventive counseling, and educational services on the topic of pregnancy for teenagers:

- DC CAMPAIGN TO PREVENT TEEN PREGNANCY
  1112 Eleventh Street, NW, Suite 100
  Washington, DC 20001
  Phone: 202-789-4666
  Website: http://www.teenpregnancydc.org

- THE NATIONAL CAMPAIGN TO PREVENT TEEN AND UNPLANNED PREGNANCY
  1776 Massachusetts Avenue, NW, Suite 200
  Washington, DC 20036

APPENDIX X

PROGRAMS FOR THE PREVENTION AND TREATMENT OF JUVENILE DELINQUENCY

NATIONAL INSTITUTE OF MENTAL HEALTH
Science Writing, Press and Dissemination Branch
6001 Executive Boulevard
Room 8184, MSC 0663
Bethesda, MD 20892-9663

Phone: 1-866-615-6464 (toll-free)
E-mail: nimhinfo@nih.gov
Web site: http://www.nimh.nih.gov

APPENDIX XI

THE DSM-IV-TR MULTIAXIAL SYSTEM OF DIAGNOSIS

There are five axes included in the DSM-IV-TR multiaxial classification. Each axis refers to a different domain of information related to the patient's presenting problems.

Axis I   Clinical Disorders
         Other Conditions That May Be a Focus of Clinical Attention
Axis II   Personality Disorders
         Mental Retardation
Axis III General Medical Conditions
Axis IV Psychosocial and Environmental Problems
Axis V   Global Assessment of Functioning

A comprehensive evaluation necessitates addressing all five axes. Psychiatric disorders other than personality disorders and mental retardation are listed on Axis I. Examples are: Mood disorders and Anxiety disorders. Sometimes patients will seek out mental health services even if they do not suffer from a psychiatric disorder. Examples are: marital problems and bereavement. Such conditions are also reported on Axis I. Personality Disorders and Mental Retardation are listed on Axis II. Examples are: Borderline Personality Disorder and Moderate Mental Retardation. General Medical Conditions are reported on Axis III. Examples are: Epilepsy and Chronic Pulmonary Heart Disease. Psychosocial and environmental problems or stressors that relate to a person's clinical disorder are listed on Axis IV. Examples are: sexual or physical abuse, discrimination, illiteracy, and extreme poverty. The patient's overall psychological, social and occupational level of functioning is listed on Axis V. Examples are: gross impairment in communication, inability to maintain minimal personal hygiene, and severe obsessional rituals.

This multiaxial system is useful not only for clinical evaluation, but also for proper treatment planning and for realistic treatment expectations. (American Psychiatric Association, 2000)

APPENDIX XII

SUPPORT GROUPS AND ORGANIZATIONS RELATED TO CHILDHOOD PSYCHIATRIC DISORDERS

NATIONAL INSTITUTE OF MENTAL HEALTH
Science Writing, Press and Dissemination Branch
6001 Executive Boulevard
Room 8184, MSC 6993
Bethesda, MD 20892-9663

Phone: 1-866-615-6464
E-mail: nimhinfo@nih.gov
Web site: http://www.nimh.nih.gov

Local city and state mental health organizations are also available for information.

APPENDIX XIII

FACTORS ASSOCIATED WITH SUICIDE RISK
IN CHILDREN AND ADOLESCENTS

- *Gender.* While girls are more likely than boys to attempt suicide, boys are more likely to succeed in their attempts.

- *Geography.* Adolescents in rural, less populated areas are more likely to commit suicide.

- *Ethnicity.* Suicide rate is higher in non-Hispanic white youth than in African American, Asian American and Hispanic American youth. Suicide rate is high among Native American young adults.

- *Depression, hopelessness and low self-esteem.* Depression, combined with feelings of hopelessness and low self-esteem are often predictors of suicidal thoughts and acts.

- *Previous suicidal behavior.* Adolescents with a history of suicide attempts are at high risk; those who talk about death or suicidal ideas, or engage in dangerous behaviors are also at risk. Teenage suicide is more frequent where there is a family history of suicide.

- *Prior sexual abuse.* A history of childhood sexual abuse increases the probability of suicidal behavior in late adolescence.

- *Family problems.* Exposure to a stressful and problematic family environment, such as physical abuse, death of a parent, divorce, neglectful parental attitude, and ineffective parent-child communication are associated with suicidal behavior.

- *Stressful life events.* Traumatic and stressful life events often precipitate suicidal plans or acts. Examples of such events are legal problems, interruption of a romantic relationship, unwanted pregnancy, or academic problems.

- *Substance abuse.* Drug or alcohol addiction in the family, or by the adolescent increases the likelihood for suicide.

- *Social contagion.* When suicidal acts by a group or an individual gets widespread publicity, others may become "infected" with the idea of self-destruction, and adopt such behavior as a preferred means of dealing with pressures and the stresses of life (Pelkonen & Marttunen, 2003).

APPENDIX XIV

RECOMMENDATIONS FOR SUICIDE PREVENTION

The following guidelines may prove useful when faced with a person who talks about or threatens suicide:

1. *Recognize the seriousness of the situation.* While it is true that some people who talk about suicide may "not really mean it", it is a big mistake to minimize the seriousness of suicidal intentions. Whoever talks about suicide must be taken seriously!

2. *Implied threats must be taken seriously.* Not everyone talks about suicide in a direct fashion. Allusions such as "life is not worth living", or "I wish not to wake up in the morning" must be taken seriously.

3. *Express understanding.* Make the person feel that you are aware of their concerns, and that you care about their emotional state. Avoid statements such as "we all feel depressed at times", or "time will heal such feelings".

4. *Focus on alternatives.* Suggest to the person that there are many other approaches to solve the person's problems, even if such solutions may not be presently apparent.

5. *Assess the immediate danger.* Ask the person if he/she has any plans in mind regarding the mode of suicide. If drugs, guns or hanging are mentioned, prevent the person from going home alone. If jumping from tall buildings or bridges are mentioned, prevent the person from being alone.

6. *Enlist the person's agreement to seek help.* Make every attempt to have the person accompany you to a hospital emergency room, or to a health professional. Explain to the person that professional help is available, effective, and is presently needed. If necessary, call a health professional or a suicide help line at 1-800-SUICIDE.

7. *Accompany the person to seek help.* The suicidal person should never be left alone. If the person refuses help, call the police for assistance (Nevid, Rathus, & Greene, 2011).

APPENDIX XV

BEHAVIORAL EFFECTS OF BLOOD ALCOHOL LEVELS

Percentage of blood alcohol concentration	**Behavioral effects**
.05	Lowered alertness; release of inhibitions; impaired judgment
.10	Slowed reaction times; impaired motor function; less caution
.15	Large, consistent decreases in reaction time
.20	Marked depression in sensory and motor capability; decidedly intoxicated
.25	Severe motor disturbance; staggering; sensory perceptions greatly impaired
.30	Stuporous but conscious; no comprehension of the external world
.35	Condition equivalent to surgical anesthesia; minimal level at which death occurs
.40	Death in about 50 percent of cases

(Ray & Ksir, 1990)

APPENDIX XVI

RESOURCES RELATED TO COGNITIVE DISORDERS

Alzheimer's Foundation of America
322 8th Avenue 7th floor
New York, N.Y. 10001
Phone: 1-866-AFA-8484

Alzheimer's Association
225 N. Michigan Avenue
Chicago, Illinois 60601-7633
Phone: 1-800-272-3900
E-mail: info@ALZ.ORG

National Institute on Aging
Alzheimer's Disease Education and Referral Center
HTTP://WWW.NIA.NIH.GOV/ALZHEIMERS

Brain Injury Association of America
1608 Spring Hill Road Suite 110
Vienna, VA 22182
Phone: 703-761-0750
800-444-6443

National Institute of Health
Neurological Institute
P.O.Box 5801
Bethesda, MD 20824
Phone: 800-352-9424
301-496-5751

APPENDIX XVII

FREQUENTLY USED TESTS IN PSYCHIATRIC HOSPITALS, CLINICS, AND IN PRIVATE CLINICAL PSYCHOLOGY PRACTICES

Wechsler Adult Intelligence Scale-Revised (WAIS-IV)*
(General intellectual functioning in adults)

Wechsler Intelligence Scale for Children-Revised (WISC-R and III)*
(General intellectual functioning in children)

Minnesota Multiphasic Personality Inventory (MMPI) I and II*
(Personality characteristics suggestive of adult and adolescent psychopathology)

Rorschach Inkblot Test
(Personality dynamics including characteristics of perception)

Bender Visual Motor Gestalt Test*
(Spatial abilities)

Thematic Apperception Test (TAT)
(Identification of dominant emotions, conflicts, needs, and complexes in adults)

Children's Apperception Test (CAT)
(Identification of anxieties, conflicts, and feelings of guilt in children)

Wide Range Achievement Test-R and III (WRAT)*
(Basic skills in arithmetic, spelling, and reading)

House-Tree-Person Projective Technique
(Personality and emotional characteristics, including self-concept, and perceptions related to family dynamics)

Wechsler Memory Scale-Revised (WMS-R)*
(Global and specific memory functions)

Beck Depression Inventory (BDI)
(Symptoms and severity of depression)

Trail Making Test A and B*
(Attentional functions)

FAS Word Fluency Test*
(Fluency of speech)

Halstead-Reitan Neuropsychological Test Battery*
(Integrity of general cognitive functions)

Boston Memory Test*
(Verbal memory)

Category Test*
(Visual concept formation and abstraction)

( )Items in parentheses describe the function of tests.
*Tests which may be used for the identification and measurement of brain damage.

COMMONLY USED PSYCHOTROPIC MEDICATIONS

Antidepressants

Tricyclics

†Anafranil (clomipramine)
Asendin (amoxapine)
Elavil (amitriptyline)
Norpramin (desipramine)
Pamelor (nortriptyline)
Sinequan (doxepin)
Surmontil (trimipramine)
Tofranil (imipramine)
Vivactil (protiptyline)

*Common side effects of tricyclic antidepressants include: dry mouth, drowsiness, lightheadedness, confusion, tremors, dizziness, headaches, constipation, ejaculation failure, blurred vision, difficulty urinating.

Selective Serotonin Reuptake Inhibitors (SSRIs)

Celexa (citalopram)
Lexapro (escitalopram)
†Luvox (fluvoxamine)
†Paxil (paroxetine)
†Prozac (fluoxetine)
†Zoloft (sertraline)

†These medications are also used for the treatment of obsessive compulsive disorder.

*Common side effects of SSRI antidepressants include: nausea, dry mouth, insomnia, headache, fatigue, ejaculation problems, weakness, drowsiness, diarrhea, loss of appetite, anxiety, weight loss, erectile dysfunction, decreased sex drive.

Monoamine Oxidase Inhibitors (MAOIs)

Nardil (phenelzine)
Parnate (tranylcypromate)

*Common side effects of MAOI antidepressants include: dizziness, drowsiness, insomnia, fatigue, twitching, constipation, dry mouth, weight gain, fluid retention, low blood pressure, ejaculation problems, erectile dysfunction.

Miscellaneous Antidepressants

Desyrel (trazadone)
Effexor (venlafaxine)
Remeron (mirtazapine)
Serzone (nefazodone)
Wellbutrin (bupropion)

*Common side effects of miscellaneous antidepressants include: dry mouth drowsiness, dizziness, lightheadedness, nausea, headaches, insomnia, nervousness, loss or increase of appetite, weakness, sweating, high cholesterol, weight gain, tremors, vomiting.

Mood Stabilizers (used in the treatment of bipolar disorder)

Depakene (valproic acid)
Depakote (devalproex)
Eskalith
Lithobid (lithium)
Lithonate

Lithotabs
‡Lamictal (lamotrigine)
‡Neurontin (gabapentin)
‡Tegretol (carbamazepine)
‡Topamax (topiramate)
•Zyprexa (olanzapine)
•Seroquel (quetiapine)
•Abilify (aripiprazole)
•Geodon (ziprasidone)

•Also used for the treatment of psychotic disorders
*Common side effects of mood stabilizers include: weight loss or gain, hair loss, kidney problems, nausea, tremor, water retention, skin rash, diarrhea, dry mouth, constipation, dizziness, sleepiness, fatigue, nervousness, coordination problems, confusion, loss of appetite, development of diabetes, disturbances in menstrual functioning, breast milk secretion, headaches, restlessness, heartburn, respiratory infection.

Anti-Panic Agents

Klonopin (clonazepam)
Paxil (paroxetine)

*Common side effects of anti-panic agents include: drowsiness, confusion, slurred speech, dizziness, fatigue, memory problems, headaches, constipation, dry mouth, insomnia, nausea, ejaculation problems.

<u>Antianxiety Agents</u>

Ativan (lorazepam)
BuSpar (buspirone
Centrax (prazepam)

‡Inderal (propranolol)
‡Klonopin (clonazepam)
Lexapro (escitalopram)
Librium (chlordiazepoxide)
Serax (oxazepam)
‡Tenormin (atenolol)
Tranxene (clorazepate)
Valium (diazepam)
Xanax (alprazolam)

‡These are antidepressant medications, also used in the treatment of anxiety.

*Common side effects of antianxiety agents include: nausea, headaches, dizziness, drowsiness, upset stomach, constipation, diarrhea, dry mouth, clumsiness, sleepiness, erectile dysfunction, fatigue, lightheadedness, slurry speech, disorientation, confusion, slow reflexes, impaired thinking and judgement, memory loss.

Antipsychotics (used in the treatment of schizophrenia and mania)

Typical Antipsychotics

Haldol (haloperidol)
Loxitane (loxapine)
Mellaril (thioridazine)
Moban (molindone)
Navane (thiothixene)
Prolixin (fluphenazine)
Serentil (mesoridazine)
Stelazine (trifluoperazine)
Thorazine (chlorpromazine)
Trilafon (perphenazine)

Clozapin (clozaril)

*Common side effects of typical antipsychotics include: dry mouth, tremor, leukopenia, aggranulocytosis (reduction in white blood cells), tardive dyskinesia (severe involuntary movement disorder), seizure, disturbances in temperature regulation, eczema, salivation, low blood pressure, dizziness, rapid heart rate, drawsiness, light sensitivity, skin irritations, lactation, menstrual irregularities, hypo/hyperglycemia, nausea, anorexia, diarrhea, constipation, erectile dysfunction, ejaculation problems, urine retention, blurred vision.

Atypical Antipsychotics

Abilify (aripiprazole)
Clorazil (clozapine)
Geodon (ziprasidone)
Risperdal (risperidone)
Seroquel (quetiapine)
Zyprexa (olanzapine)

*Side effects are listed under mood stabilizers.

Stimulants (used in the treatment of ADHD)

Adderal (amphetamine/dextroamphetamine)
Cylert (pemoline)
Dexedrine (dextroamphetamine)
Ritalin (methylphenidate)

*Common side effects of stimulants include: loss of appetite, dry mouth, insomnia, headaches, stomach pain, weight loss, nausea, vomiting, emotional changes, weakness, elevated heart rate, urinary tract infection, fever, heartburn, elevated blood pressure, skin rash, restlessness, liver dysfunction, movement disorder, depression, dizziness, eye movement problems, changes in blood glucose.

*Severity of side effects may depend on individuals' tolerance for drugs. Risks related to medication side effects should always be discussed with the prescribing physician. Pregnant women need to consult their gynecologists before ingesting any medication. Medication interactions, allergies, and interaction of medications with certain food products also need to be discussed. Pharmacists may also be consulted regarding necessary precautions and safety of drugs.

The above list of brand and generic names of medications were provided by the National Alliance on Mental Illness (NAMI).

It is important to consult your psychiatrist
regarding the above information!

APPENDIX XIX

EXAMPLES OF BOOKS FOR CHILDREN
ABOUT PREGNANCY AND CHILDBIRTH

Waiting for Baby by Harriet Ziefert

Baby on the Way by William Sears, M.D., Martha Sears, R.N., and Christie Watts Kelly

Additional books and related literature may be obtained from pediatricians, child psychologists, local libraries and bookstores.

APPENDIX XX

INFORMATION SOURCES ABOUT
CAREER GUIDANCE FOR ADULTS

AMERICAN PSYCHOLOGICAL ASSOCIATION
750 First Avenue N.E.
Washington, D.C. 20002-4242

Phone: 800-3742721; 202-336-5500

U.S. DEPARTMENT OF LABOR
Frances Perkins Building
200 Constitution Avenue N.W.
Washington, D.C. 20210

Phone: 1-866-487-2365
Web site: www.dol.gov

Further information may be obtained from local city, state, and private social service agencies. Industrial psychologists may also be consulted.

INFORMATION RELATED TO THE CARE OF
SICK AND ELDERLY INDIVIDUALS

FAMILY CAREGIVER ALLIANCE
National Center on Caregiving
National Family Caregivers Association

Contact: info@caregiver.org

BRAIN INJURY ASSOCIATION OF AMERICA
1608 Spring Hills Road, Suite 110
Vienna, VA. 22182

Phone: 703-761-0750

NATIONAL PARKINSON FOUNDATION, INC.
1501 N.W. 9th Avenue/Bob Hope Road
Miami, Florida 33136-1494

Phone: 1-800-327-4545
Contact: contact@parkinson.org

AMERICAN STROKE ASSOCIATION
7272 Greenville Avenue
Dallas, Texas 75231

Phone: 1-888-478-7653

ELDER HELPERS

Phone: 734-330-2734

Contact: help@elderhelpers.org

Further information may also be obtained at local city and state departments of the aging, and departments

APPENDIX XXII

SOURCES OF INFORMATION RELATED TO RETIREMENT OPTIONS

U.S. DEPARTMENT OF HEALTH AND HUMAN SERVICES
200 Independence Avenue S.W.
Washington, D.C. 20201

Phone: 1-877-696-6775
Web site: www.hhs.gov

ALLIANCE FOR RETIRED AMERICANS
815 16th Street N.W.
Fourth Floor
Washington, D.C. 20006

Phone: 202-637-5399

AMERICAN ASSOCIATION OF RETIRED PERSONS
Web site: www.aarp.org

NEW YORK STATE DEPARTMETNT OF THE AGING
Senior Citizen's Help Line: 1-800-342-9871

GAY AND LESBIAN ASSOCIATION OF RETIRING PERSONS, INC.
10940 Wilshire Boulevard Suite 1600
Los Angeles, CA 90024

Phone: 310-722-1807; 310-477-0707
Contact: glarpinc@gmail.com

CANADIAN ASSOCIATION OF RETIRED PERSONS
30 Jefferson Avenue
Toronto, ON M6K 1Y4
Canada

Phone: 888-363-2279
Contact: support@carp.ca

APPENDIX XXIII

INFORMATION SOURCES RELATED TO CHILD AND ADOLESCENT MENTAL DISORDERS

NATIONAL ALLIANCE ON MENTAL ILLNESS (NAMI)
3803 N. Fairfax Drive, Suite 100
Arlington, VA 22203

Phone: 703-524-7600; 1-800-950-6264

NATIONAL INSTITUTE OF MENTAL HEALTH (NIMH)
6001 Executive Boulevard
Rm. 8184, MSC 9663
Bethesda, MD 20892-9663

Phone: 1-866-615-6464
Web site: www.nimh.nih.gov

Information may also be obtained from local city and state departments of mental health.

APPENDIX XXIV

INFORMATION SITE RELATED TO
LEARNING DISABILITIES

LEARNING DISABILITIES ASSOCIATION OF AMERICA
4146 Library Road
Pittsburgh, PA 15234-1349

Phone: 412-341-1515

Further information may be obtained from local city and state departments of mental health and departments of education.

APPENDIX XXV

SELF-HELP ORGANIZATIONS FOR ALCOHOLISM AND SUBSTANCE ABUSE DISORDERS

ALCOHOLICS ANONYMOUS
Web site: www.aa.org
Telephone directories may be used for a listing of local chapters.

AL-ANON AND ALATEEN FAMILY GROUPS
Phone: 888-425-2666

NAR-ANON FAMILY GROUPS
Web site: www.nar-anon.org

Telephone directories may be used for a listing of local chapters.

APPENDIX XXVI

INFORMATION SOURCES RELATED
TO EATING DISORDERS

NATIONAL INSTITUTE OF MENTAL HEALTH (NIMH)
6001 Executive Boulevard
Room 8184, MSC 9663
Bethesda, MD 20892-9663

Phone: 1-866-615-6464
Web site: www.nih.gov

NATIONAL EATING DISORDERS ASSOCIATION (NEDA)
165 W 46th Street
New York, N.Y. 10036

Help line: 800-931-2237
Phone: 212-575-6200

NATIONAL ASSOCIATION OF ANOREXIA NERVOSA AND
ASSOCIATED DISORDERS, INC.
800 E. Diehl Road #160
Naperville, Illinois 60563

Help line: 630-577-1330
Phone: 630-577-1333
Contact: anadhelp@anad.org

REFERENCES

Aguiar, A., & Baillargeon, R. (2002). Developments in young infants reasoning about occluded objects. Cognitive Psychology, 45 (2), 267-336.

Aiken, L.R. (2003). Psychological testing and assessment (11th ed.) Boston, MA: Allyn and Bacon.

Aiken, L.R. & Groth-Marnat, G. (2006). Psychological Testing and Assessment (12th ed.). Boston: Allyn and Bacon.

Ainsworth, M.D.S., & Bowlby, K. (1991). An ethnological approach to personality development. American Psychologist, 46 (4), 333-341.

Amato, P.R. (2006). Marital discord, divorce and children's well-being. Results from a 20-year longitudinal study of two generations. In A. Clarke-Stewart and J. Dunn (Eds.), Families count: Effects on child and adolescent development. The Jacobs Foundation series on adolescence (pp. 179-202). New York: Cambridge University Press.

American Academy of Family Physicians (2006, November 1). Nutrition in toddlers. American Family Physician, 74 (9).

American Academy of Pediatrics (2003). Policy statement. Pediatrics, 112, (2), 424-430.

American Psychiatric Association. (2000). DSM-IV-TR: Diagnostic and statistical manual of mental disorders (4th ed., Text-Revision) Washington, DC: Author.

Annett, M. (1999). Left-handedness as a function of sex, maternal versus paternal inheritance, and report bias. Behavior Genetics 29 (2), 103-114.

Annett, M., and Moran, P. (2006). Schizotypy is increased in mixed-handers, especially right-handed writers who use the left hand for primary actions. Schizophrenia Research, 81 (2-3), 239-246.

Apgar, V. (1953). A proposal for a new method of evaluation in the newborn infant. Current Research in Anesthesia and Analgesia, 32, 260-267.

Bale, J.F.J. (2002) Congenital infections. Neurological Clinic, 20 (4), 1039-1060.

Barlow, D.H. and Durand, V.M. (2005). Abnormal Psychology: An Integrative Approach. (4th ed.). Belmont, CA: Thomson Wadsworth.

Bauman, M.L., Anderson, G., Perry, E. & Ray, M. (2006). Neuroanatomical and neurochemical studies of the autistic brain: Current thought and future directions. In S.O. Moldin & J.L.R. Rubenstein (Eds.), Understanding autism: From basic neuroscience to treatment (pp. 303-322). Boca Raton, FL: CRC Press.

Baumrind, D. (1989). Rearing competent children. In W. Damon (Ed.), Child development today and tomorrow. San Francisco: Jossey-Bass.

Bayley, N. (1969). Bayley Scales of Infant Development. New York: Psychological Corporation.

Beck, A.T. (1967). Depression: causes and treatment. Philadelphia: University of Pennsylvania Press.

Behnke, S.H., Perlin, M.L., and Bernstein, M. (2003). The essentials of New York mental health law: A straightforward guide for clinicians of all disciplines. New York, N.Y.: Norton.

Belsky, J. (2001). Emanuel Miller Lecture: Developmental risks (still) associated with child care. Journal of Child Psychology and Psychiatry, 42, 845-859.

Belsky, J. (2006). Determinants and consequences of infant-parent attachment. In L. Balter & C.S. Tamis-Lemonda (Eds.), Child psychology & A handbook of contemporary issues (2nd ed.) (pp. 53-77). New York: Psychology Press.

Belsky, J. (2006). Early childcare and early child development: Major findings of the NICHD Study of Early Child Care. European Journal of Developmental Psychology 3, (1), 95-110.

Bendersky, M. & Lewis, M. (1998) Arousal modulation in cocaine-exposed infants. Developmental Psychology, 3, 555-564.

Bengtson, H. (2005). Children's cognitive appraisal of others' distressful and positive experiences. International Journal of Behavioral Development, 29, 457-466.

Bernstein, D.P., and Travaglini, L. (1999). Schizoid and avoidant personality disorders. In T. Millon, P.H. Blaney, and R.D. Davis (Eds.), Oxford textbook of psychopathology (pp. 523-534). New York: Oxford University Press.

Berk, L.E. (2010). Development Through the Lifespan (5th ed.). Boston, MA: Allyn & Bacon.

Berk, L.E. (2013). <u>Child Development</u> (9th ed.). Upper Saddle River, New Jersey: Pearson.

Bigner, J.J. (2010). <u>Parent-Child Relations: An Introduction to Parenting</u> (8th ed.). Upper Saddle River, New Jersey: Merrill.

Birmaher, B., Axelson, D., Strober, M., Bill, M.K., Valeri, S., Chiappetta, L., et. al. (2006). Clinical course of children and adolescents with bipolar disorders. <u>Archives of General Psychiatry, 63</u>, 175-183.

Bloom, L. (1998) Language acquisition in its developmental context. In W. Daman (Ed.), <u>Handbook of child psychology</u> (5th ed.), Vol. 2. New York: Wiley.

Boccia, M. & Campos, J.J. (1989) Maternal emotional signals, social referencing and infants' reactions to strangers. In N/ Eisenberg (Ed.), New directions for child development, No. 44. <u>Empathy and related emotional responses</u>. San Francisco: Jossey-Bass.

Booth-LaForce, C., et. al. (2006). Attachment, self-worth, and peer-group functioning in middle childhood. <u>Attachment and Human Development, 8</u> (4), 309-325.

Brazelton, T.B. (1973). <u>Neonatal Behavioral Assessment Scale</u> (Clinics in Developmental Medicine, No. 50). Philadelphia, PA: J.B. Lippincott.

Brazelton, T.B., & Nugent, J.K. (1995). <u>Neonatal Behavioral Assessment Scale</u>. London, MacKeith Press.

Brennan, J.F. (2003). <u>History and systems of psychology</u> (6th ed.). Upper Saddle River, N.J.: Prentice Hall.

Bridges, K. (1932). Emotional development in early infancy. <u>Child Development, 3</u>, 324-341.

Brown, R., and Fraser, C. (1963). The acquisition of syntax. In C.N. Cofer and B. Musgrave (Eds.). <u>Verbal behavior and learning: Problems and processes.</u> New York: McGraw Hill.

Bryden, P.J., Broyn, J., and Fletcher, P. (2005). Handedness and health: An examination of the association between different handedness classifications and health disorders. <u>Laterality: Asymmetries of Body, Brain, and Cognition, 10</u> (5), 429-440.

Bushnell, I.W.R. (2001) Mother's face recognition in newborn infants: Learning and memory. <u>Infant and Child Development, 10</u> (1-2), 67-74.

Butcher, J.N., Mineka, S., & Hooley, J.M. (2007) <u>Abnormal Psychology</u> (13th ed.) Boston: Allyn and Bacon.

Calhoun, F., and Warren, K. (2007). Fetal alcohol syndrome: Historical perspectives. <u>Neurscience and Biobehavioral Reviews, 31,</u> 168-171.

Care Study Group. (2008). Maternal caffeine intake during pregnancy and risk of fetal growth restriction: A large prospective observational study. <u>British Medical Journal, 337,</u> a2337.

Caton, D., Corry, M.P., Frigoletto, F.D., Hokins, D.P., Liberman, E., & Mayberry, L. (2002). The nature and management of labor pain: Executive summary. <u>American Journal of Obstetrics and Gynecology, 186,</u> S1-S15.

Chamberlain, P., and Reid, J.B. (1998). Comparison of two community alternatives to incarceration for chronic juvenile offenders. Journal of Consulting and Clinical Psychology, 66 (4), 624-633.

Chan, A., Keane, R.J., & Robinson, J.S. (2001). The contribution of maternal smoking to preterm birth, small for gestational age and low birth weight among Aboriginal and non-Aboriginal births in South Australia. Medical Journal of Australia, 174 (8),389-393.

Chaukin, W. (1995). Substance abuse in pregnancy. In B.P. Sachs, R. Beard, E.Papiernik, & C. Russell (Eds.), Reproductive health care for women and babies (pp. 305-321). New York: Oxford University Press.

Chertok, I., Luo, J., & Anderson, R.H. (2011). Association between changes in smoking habits in subsequent pregnancy and infant birthweight in West Virginia. Maternal and Child Health Journal, 15, 249-254.

Christian, P. (2002). Maternal nutrition, health, and survival. Nutritional Review, 60, 559-563.

Clark, E.A., and Hanisee, J. (1982). Intellectual and adaptive performance of Asian children in adoptive settings. Developmental Psychology, 18, 595-599.

Clark, K.E., & Ladd, G.W. (2000). Connectedness and autonomy support in parent-child relationships: Links to children's socioemotional orientation and peer relationships. Developmental Psychology, 36 (4), 485-498.

Claxton, L.J., Keen, R., & McCarty, M.E. (2003). Evidence of motor planning in infant reading behavior. Psychological Science, 14, 354-356.

Cole, M., Cole, S.R., & Lightfoot, C. (2005). The Development of Children (5th ed.). New York: Worth Publishers.

Coley, R.L., and Chase-Lansdale, P.L. (1998). Adolescent pregnancy and parenthood. Recent evidence and future directions. American Psychologist, 5. (2), 152-166.

Cook, E.H. (1990). Autism: Review of neurochemical investigation. Synapse, 6, 292-308.

Coren, S. (1992). The left-hander syndrome. New York: Free Press.

Costello, E.J., Egger, H., & Angold, A. (2005). Ten-year research update review: The epidemiology of child and adolescent psychiatric disorders: I. Methods and public health burden. Journal of the American Academy of Child & Adolescent Psychiatry, 44, 972-986.

Craig, C., and Sprang, G. (2007). Trauma exposure and child abuse potential: Investigating the cycle of violence. American Journal of Orthopsychiatry, 77, (2), 296-305.

Crowl, A., Ahn, S, & Baker, J. (2008). A meta-analysis of developmental outcomes for children of same-sex and heterosexual parents. Journal of GLBT Family Studies, 4, 385-407.

Cunningham, F.G., MacDonald P.C., Grant, N.F., Leveno, K.J., Gilstrap, L.C., III, Hankins, G.D.V., & Clark, S.L. (2001) Williams obstetrics (21st ed.) Stamford, CT: Appleton & Lange.

Dales, L., Hammer, S.J., & Smith, N.J. (2001). Time trends in autism and MMR immunization coverage in California. Journal of the American Medical Association, 285, 1183-1185.

Daniels, S.R. (2006). The consequences of childhood overweight and obesity. The Future of Children, 16 (1), 47-67.

Davies, P.T., and Cummings, E.M. (1998). Exploring children's emotional insecurity as a mediator of the link between marital relations and child adjustment. Child Development, 69, 124-139.

Devi, N.P.G., Shenbagvalli, R., Ramesh, K., & Rathinam, S.N. (2009). Rapid progression of HIV infection in infancy. Indian Pediatrics, 46, 63-56.

de Zwaan, M. (2003). Basic neuroscience and scanning. In J. Treasure, V. Schmidt, and E. Van Furth (Eds.) Handbook of Eating Disorders, 2e (pp.89-101). Hoboken, NJ: John Wiley & Sons.

Domino, G. and Domino, M.L. (2006). Psychological testing: An introduction. (2nd ed.). New York, N.Y.: Cambridge University Press.

Dougall, A.L. & Baum, A. (2001). Stress, health, and illness. In A. Baum, T.A. Revenson, & J.E. Singer (Eds.). Handbook of health psychology (pp. 321-337). Mahwah, N.J.: Erlbaum.

Dunn, J., and Hughes, C. (2001). "I got some swords and you're dead!" Violent fantasy, antisocial behavior, friendship, and moral sensibility in young children. Child Development, 72 (2), 491-505.

Eckenrode, J., Laird, M., & Doris, J. (1993). School performance and disciplinary problems among abused and neglected children. Developmental Psychology, 29; 53-62.

Eliez, S., Blasey, C.M., Freund, L.S., Hastie, T., and Reiss, A.L. (2001). Brain anatomy, gender, and IQ in children and adolescents with fragile X syndrome. Brain, 124, 1610-1618.

Ellis, B. J. (2004). Timing of pubertal maturation in girls: An integrated life history approach. Psychological Bulletin, 130, 920-958.

Englund, M.M., Levy, A.K., Hyson, D.M., & Sroufe, L.A. (2000). Adolescent social competence: Effectiveness in a group setting. Child Development, 71, 1049-1060.

Ewen, R.B. (2003) An Introduction to theories of personality (6th ed.). Mahwah, NJ: Lawrence Erlbaum Associates.

Fantz, R.L. (1961). The origins of form perception. Scientific American 204 (5) 66-72.

Feldman, R.S. (2012). Child Development. (6th ed.). Upper Saddle River, New Jersey: Pearson.

Fischer, L., Ames, E.W., Chisholm, K., & Savoie, L. (1997). Problems reported by parents of Romanian orphans adopted to British Columbia. International Journal of Behavioral Development, 20, 67-82.

Fivush, R., Kuebli, J., & Clubb, P.A. (1992). The structure of events and event representations: A developmental analysis. Child Development, 63, 188-201.

Foley, G.M. (2006). Self and social-emotional development in infancy: A descriptive synthesis. In G.M. Foley & J.D. Hochman (Eds.), Mental Health in early intervention: Achieving unity in principles and practice (pp.139- 173). Baltimore: Paul H. Brookes.

Franklin, M.E., Aramowitz, J.S., Kozak, M.J., Levitt, J.T, et.al. (2000). Effectiveness of exposure and ritual prevention for obsessive-compulsive disorder: Randomized compared with nonrandomized samples. Journal of Consulting and Clinical Psychology, 68, 594-602.

Friedman, J.M. & Polifka, J.E. (1996). The effects of drugs on the fetus and nursing infants. Baltimore: John Hopkins University Press.

Gardner, H. (1983). Frames of mind: The theory of multiple intelligences. New York: Basic Books.

Gartstein, M.A., Slobodskaya, H.R., & Kinsht, I.A. (2003). Cross-cultural differences in temperament in the first year of life: United States of America (U.S.) and Russia. International Journal of Behavioral Development, 27 (4), 316-328.

Ghetti, S., and Alexander, K.W. (2004). "If it happened, I would remember it": Strategic use of event memorability in the rejection of false autobiographical events. Child Development, 75 (2), 542-561.

Gibbs, J.C., Potter, G.B., DiBiase, A.-M., & Devlin, R. (2009). The EQUIP program: Social perspective-taking for responsible thought and behavior. In B. Glick. (Ed.), Cognitive behavioral interventions for at-risk youth (2nd ed.). Kingston, N.J.: Civic Research Institute.

Gibson, E.J., & Walker, A.S. (1984). Development of knowledge of visual-tactile affordances of substance. Child Development, 55, 453-460.

Gleitman, L., and Landau, B. (1994). The acquisition of the lexicon. Cambridge, MA: Bradford.

Goddard, A.W., Mason, G.F., Almai, A., Rothman, D.L., Behar, K.L., et. al. (2001). Reductions in occipital cortex GABA levels in panic disorder detected with ¹h-magnetic spectroscopy. Archives of General Psychiatry, 58, 556-561.

Godfrey, K.W., & Barker, D.J.P. (2000). Fetal nutrition and adult disease. American Journal of Clinical Nutrition, 71 (Suppl. 5), 13445-13525.

Golden, C.J., Purisch, A.D., & Hammeke, T.A. (1985). Luria-Nebraska Neuropsychological Battery: Forms I and II. Los Angeles: Western Psychological Services.

Golub, S. (1992). Periods: From menarche to menopause. Newbury Park, CA: Sage.

Green, K.E. (1991). Measurement theory. In K.E. Green (Ed.) Educational testing: Issues and applications (pp. 3-25). New York: Garland Publishing.

Greene, E., Heilbrun, K, Fortune, W.H., and Nietzel, M.T. (2007). Wrightsman's psychology and the legal system. (6th ed.). Belmont, CA: Wadsworth.

Grusec, J.E. (2002). Parenting socialization and children's acquisition of values. In M. H. Bornstein (Ed.), Handbook of parenting (2nd ed.), Vol. 5, Practical issues in parenting (pp. 143-167). Mahwah, NJ: Erlbaum.

Hansell, J. and Damour, L. (2008). Abnormal Psychology (2nd ed.). Hoboken, New Jersey: Wiley.

Hartup, W.W. (1993). Adolescents and their friends. In B. Laursen (Ed.). New directions in child development. no. 60, Close friendships in adolescence. San Francisco: Jossey-Bass.

Hergenhahn, B.R. (2009). An introduction to the history of psychology (6th ed.). Belmont, CA: Wadsworth.

Hergenhahn, B.R. and Olson, M.H. (2007). An introduction to theories of personality (7th ed.). Upper Saddle River, NJ: Pearson/ Prentice Hall.

Hetherington, E.M., Bridges, M., & Insabella, G.M. (1998). What matters, what does not? Five perspectives on the association between marital transitions and children's adjustment. American Psychologist, 53, 167-184.

Hill, S.W., & Flom, R. (2007). 18-and 24-month-olds' discrimination of gender-consistent and inconsistent activities. Infant Behavior and Development, 30 (1) 168-173.

Hinojosa, T., Shev, C-F., & Michael, G.F. (2003). Infant hand-use preference for grasping objects contributes to the development of a hand-use preference for manipulating objects. Developmental Psychobiology, 43, 328-334.

Hoff, E. (2006). Language experience and language milestones during early childhood. In K. McCartney & D. Philips (Eds.), Blackwell handbook of early childhood development. Blackwell handbooks of developmental psychology (pp. 233-251). Malden, MA: Blackwell.

Izard, C.E. (2004). The generality-specificity issue in infants' emotion responses: A comment on Bennett, Beudersky and Lewis (2002). Infancy, 6 (3), 417-423.

Jones, D.C., Swift, D.J., & Johnson, M.A. (1988). Nondeliberate memory for a novel event among preschoolers. Developmental Psychology, 24, 641-645.

Jones, J., Lopez, A., & Wilson, M. (2003). Congenital toxoplasmosis. American Family Physician, 67, 2131-2137.

Jones, R.E. (1997) Human Reproductive biology. San Diego: Academic Press.

Jorde, L.B., Carey, J.C., Bamshad, M.J. & White, R.L. (1999). Medical Genetics. St. Louis: Mosby.

Joshi, P.T., Salpekar, J.A., & Daniolos, P.T. (2006). Physical and sexual abuse of children. In M.K. Dulcan & J.M. Wiener (Eds.)., Essentials of child and adolescent psychiatry (pp. 595-620). Washington, D.C: American Psychiatric Publishing.

Kaltenbach, K., Berghella, V., Finnegan, L. & Woods, J.R., Jr. (1998). Opioid dependence during pregnancy: effects and management in substance abuse in pregnancy. Obstetrics and Gynecology Clinics of North America, 25 (1), 139-152.

Kaufman J., & Zigler, E. (1992). The prevention of child maltreatment: Programming, research, and policy. In D.J. Willis, E.W. Holden, & M. Rosenber, (Eds.), Prevention of child maltreatment: Developmental and ecological perspectives. New York: Wiley.

Kelsey, J.E., Newport, D.J., & Nemeroff, C.B. (2006). Principles of Psychopharmacology for mental health professionals. Hoboken, N.J.: Wiley-Liss.

Kiecolt-Glaser, J.K., McGuire, L., Robles, T.F., & Glaser, R. (2002). Emotion, mobility, and motality: New perspectives from psychoneuroimmunology. Ann. Rev. Psychol., 53, 83-107.

Kinsbourne, M. (2003). The corpus callosum equilibrates the cerebral hemispheres. In E. Zaidel & M. Iacoboui (Eds.) The parallel brain: The cognitive neuroscience of the corpus callosum (pp. 271-281). Cambridge, MA: MIT Press.

Kliegman, R.M., Behrman, R.E., Jenson, H.B., & Stanton, B.F. (Eds.). (2008). Nelson textbook of pediatrics e-dition. Philadelphia: Saunders.

Kohlberg, L. (1981) The meaning and measurement of moral development. Worcester, MA: Clark University Press.

Kohlberg, L. (1984). The psychology of moral development: Essays on moral development (Vol. 2). San Francisco: Harper & Row.

Kolb, B., & Gibb, R. (2007). Brain plasticity and recovery from early cortical injury. Developmental Psychobiology, 49 (2), 107-118.

Kwok, H.W.M. (2003). Psychopharmacology in autism spectrum disorders. Current Opinion in Psychiatry, 16 (5), 529-534.

Laird, R.D., Pettit, G.S., Dodge, K.A., and Bates, J.E. (2005). Peer relationship antecedents of delinquent behavior in late adolescence: Is there evidence of demographic group differences? Development and Psychopathology, 17, 127-144.

Lamb, M.E., & Ahnert, L. (2006). Nonparental child care: Context, concepts, correlates, and consequences. In K.A. Renninger, I.E. Sigel, W. Damon, & R.M. Lerner (Eds.), Handbook of child psychology (6th ed.), Vol. 4, Child psychology in practice (pp. 950-1016). Hoboken, NJ: Wiley.

Lefkowitz, E.S., and Zeldow, P.B. (2006). Masculinity and femininity predict optimal mental health: A belated test of the androgyny hypothesis. Journal of Personality Assessment, 87 (1), 95-101.

Lobel, M. (1994). Conceptualizations, measurement, and effects of prenatal maternal stress on birth outcomes. Journal of Behavioral Medicine, 17, 225-272.

Locke, J. (1699). Some thoughts concerning education (4th ed. enlarged). London: A. & J. Churchill.

Lovaas, O.I. (2003). Teaching individuals with developmental delays. Austin, TX: Pro-Ed.

Maccoby, E., and Martin, J. (1983). Socialization in the context of the family: Parent-child interaction. In E.M. Hetherington (Ed.). Handbook of child psychology: Vol. 4. Socialization, personality, and social development (pp.1-101). New York: Wiley.

Mahler, M.S., Pine, F., and Bergman, A. (1975). The psychological birth of the human infant: Symbiosis and individuation. New York: Basic Books.

Maimburg, R.D., & Vaeth, M. (2006). Perinatal risk factors and infantile autism, Acta Psychiatrica Scandinavica, 114 (4), 257-264.

Martinez, I., Musitu, G., Garcia, J.F., and Camino, L. (2003). A cross-cultural analysis of the effects of family socialization on self-concept: Spain and Brazil. Psicologia Educacion Cultura, 7 (2), 239-259.

McHale, S.M., Kim, J.-Y., and Whiteman, S.D. (2006). Sibling relationships in childhood and adolescence. In P. Noller and J.A. Feeny (Eds.), Close relationships: Functions, forms, and processes (pp.127-149). New York: Psychology Press/Taylor & Francis.

Meltzoff, A.N., & Prinz, W. (Eds.). (2002). The imitative mind: Development, evolution and brain bases. New York: Cambridge University Press.

Meyer, J.S. and Quenzer, L.F. (2005). Psychopharmacology: Drugs, the brain, and behavior. Sunderland, MA: Sinauer Associates.

Miller, C.L., Miceli, P.J., Whitman, T.L., & Borkowski, J.G. (1996). Cognitive readiness to parent and intellectual-emotional development in children of adolescent mothers. Developmental Psychology, 32, 533-541.

Minuchin, S., Rosman, B.L., & Baker, L. (1978). Psychosomatic families: Anorexia nervosa in context. Cambridge, MA: Harvard University Press.

Moore, K.L., & Persaud, T.V.N. (1993). The developing human: Clinically oriented embryology (5th ed.). Philadelphia: Saunders.

Mora, J.O., & Nestel, P.S. (2000). Improving prenatal nutrition in developing countries: Strategies, prospects, and challenges. American Journal of Clinical Nutrition, 71 (Suppl. 5), 13535-13635.

Morrell, J., & Steele, H. (2003). The role of attachment security, temperament, maternal perception, and care-giving behavior in persistent infant sleeping problems. Infant Mental Health Journal, 24 (5), 447-468.

Nelson, C.A., & Luciana, M. (Eds.). (2001). Handbook of developmental cognitive neuroscience. Cambridge, MA: MIT Press.

Nevid, J.S., Rathus, S.A., and Greene, B. (2011). Abnormal psychology in a changing world (8ᵗʰ ed.). Upper Saddle River, N.J.: Prentice Hall.

Nevid, J.S. (2013). Psychology: Concepts and Applications (4ᵗʰ ed.). California: Wadsworth.

Nevin, R. (2000). How lead exposure relates to temporal changes in IQ, violent crime, and unwed pregnancy. Environmental Research, 83, 1-22.

Patterson, C.J. (1992) Children of lesbian and gay parents. Child Development, 63, 1025-1042.

Patterson, C.J. (2003) Children of lesbian and gay parents. In L.D. Garnets and D.C. Kimmel (Eds.). Psychological perspectives on lesbian, gay and bisexual experiences (2ⁿᵈ ed.) (pp. 497-548). New York: Columbia University Press.

Paterson, R.J., and Neufeld, R.W. (1987) Clear danger: Situational determinants of the appraisal of threat. Psychological Bulletin, 101, 404-416.

Pelkonen, M., and Marttunen, M. (2003). Child and adolescent suicide: Epidemiology, risk factors, and approaches to prevention. Pediatric Drugs, 5, 243-265.

Pelphrey, K.A., et al. (2004). Development of visuospatial short-term memory in the second half of the first year. Developmental Psychology, 40 (5), 836.

Piaget, J. (1962). Play, dreams, and imitation in childhood. New York: Norton (Originally published in 1946).

Rathus, S.A. (2006). <u>Childhood and Adolescence: Voyages in Development</u> (2nd ed.) Belmont: Thomson/Wadsworth.

Rathus, S.A. (2008) <u>Childhood: Voyages in Development</u> (3rd ed.) Belmont, CA: Thomson.

Ray, O., & Ksir, C. (1990). <u>Drugs, society, and human behavior</u> (5th ed.). St. Louis: Times Mirror/Mosby.

Reed, E. (1997). The cognitive revolution from an ecological point of view. In D. M. Johnson & C.E. Erneling (Eds.), <u>The future of the cognitive revolution</u> (pp. 261-273). New York: Oxford University Press.

Reitan, R.M. & Wolfson, D. (1993). <u>The Halstead-Reitan Neuropsychological Test Battery: Theory and clinical interpretation.</u> Tucson, AZ: Neuropsychology Press.

Relier, J.-P. (2001). Influence of maternal stress on fetal behavior and brain development. <u>Biology of the Neonate</u>, 79 (3-4), 168-171.

Rice, C. (2007). Prevalence of autism spectrum disorders-Autism and Developmental Disabilities Monitoring Network, 14 Sites United States. <u>Morbidity and Mortality Weekly Report, 56</u> (5501), 12-28.

Rimoin, D.L., Connor, J.M., & Pyeritz, R.E. (1997). <u>Emery and Rimoin's principles and practice of medical genetics</u> (3rd ed.). New York: Churchill Livingstone.

Rothbart, M.K., Posner, M.I., & Hershey, K. (1995). Temperament, attention, and psychopathology. In D. Cicchetti and D. Cohen (Eds.), <u>Manual of developmental psychopathology.</u> New York: Wiley.

Rowe, D.C., Rodgers, J.L., and Meseck-Bushey,S. (1992). Sibling delinquency and the family environment: shared and unshared influences. Child Development, 63, 59-67.

Rutter, M. (2005). Genetic influences and autism. In F.R. Volkmar, R. Paul, A. Klin, & D. Cohen. (Eds.). Handbook of autism and pervasive developmental disorders (3rd ed. pp. 425-452). Hoboken, N.J.: Wiley.

Salovey, P., and Pizarro, D.A. (2003). The value of emotional intelligence. In R.J. Sternberg et. al. (Eds.), Models of intelligence: International perspectives (pp. 263-278). Washington, DC: American Psychological Association.

Sarafino, E.P. (2008). Health psychology: Biopsychosocial interactions. (6th ed.) Hoboken, N.J.: Wiley.

Selman, R.L. (1980). The growth of interpersonal understanding: Developmental and clinical analysis. New York: Academic Press.

Shaffer, D.R. (2002). Developmental psychology: Childhood and adolescence. (6th ed.). Belmont, CA: Wadsworth.

Simpson, J.L., & Golbus M.S. (1993) Genetics in obstetrics and gynecology (2nd ed.). Philadelphia: W.B. Saunders.

Smith, K.S., Cowie, H., & Blades, M. (2003). Understanding children's development. (4th ed.). pp. 222-223. Oxford: Blackwell Publishing.

Smith, M.L., Glass, G.V., and Miller, T.I. (1980). The benefits of psychotherapy. Baltimore: Johns Hopkins University Press.

Stenberg, G. (2009). Selectivity in infant social referencing. Infancy, 14, 457-473.

Sternberg, R.J. (1997). The triarchic theory of intelligence. In D.P. Flanagan, J.L. Genshaft, & P.L. Harrison (Eds.), Contemporary intellectual assessment: Theories, tests, and issues. (pp. 92-104). New York: Guilford Press.

Stevenson, R. (1977). The fetus and newly born infant: Influence of the prenatal environment (2nd ed.) St. Lois: Mosby.

Straus, M.A. (1995). Cited in C. Collins (1995, May 11), Spankings is becoming the new don't, New York Times, p. C8.

Straus, M.A., and Gelles, R.J. (Eds.). (1990). Physical violence in American families. New Brunswick, N.J.: Transaction.

Straus, M.A., and McCord, J. (1988). Do physically punished children become violent adults? In S. Nolen-Hoeksema (Ed.), Clashing views on abnormal psychology: A taking sides custom reader (pp. 130-155). Guilford, CT: Dushkin/McGraw Hill.

Strohner, H., and Nelson, K.E. (1974). The young child's development of sentence comprehension: Influence of event probability, nonverbal context, syntactic form, and strategies. Child Development, 45, 567-576.

Substance Abuse and Mental Health Services Administration Office of Applied Studies (2007). Results from the 2007 National Survey on Drug Use and Health: National findings. Rodville, MS: SAMHSA Office of Applied Studies.

Susman, E.J., Schmeelk, K.H., Ponirakia, A., & Gariepy, J.L. (2001). Maternal prenatal, postpartum, and concurrent stressors and temperament in 3-year-olds: A person and variable analysis. Development and Psychopathology, 13 (3), 629-652.

Tamis-LeMonda, C.S., Cristafaro, T.N., Rodriguez, E.T., & Bornstein, M.H. (2006) Early language development: Social influences in the first years of life. In L. Balter & C. S. Tamis-LeMonda (Eds.). Child Psychology: A handbook of contemporary issues. (2nd ed.)(pp. 79-108). New York: Psychology Press.

Thomas A., & Chess, S. (1989). Temperament and personality. In G.A. Kohnstamm, J. E. Bates, & M.K. Rothbart (Eds.), Temperament in childhood. Chichester, England: Wiley.

Thurstone, L.L., and Thurstone, T.G. (1941). Factorial studies of intelligence. Psychometric Monographs, 94 (2).

U.S. Bureau of the Census. (2004). Statistical abstract of the United States. (124th ed.). Washington, DC: U.S. Government Printing Office.

U.S. Department of Education. (2000). Trends in educational equity from girls and women. Washington, DC: Author.

U.S. Department of Health and Human Services. (2004). Child abuse and neglect fatalities: Statistics and intervention-Child Maltreatment, 2002.

Villani, S. (2001) Impact of media on children and adolescents: A 10-year review of the research. Journal of the American Academy of Child and Adolescent Psychiatry, 40 (4), 392-401.

Vorhees, C.V., and Mollnow, E. (1987). Behavioral teratogenesis: Long-term influences on behavior from early exposure to environmental agents. In J.D. Osofsky (Ed.). Handbook of Infant Development (2nd ed., pp. 913-971). New York: Wiley.

Vygotsky, L.S. (1978). Mind in society. Cambridge, MA: Harvard University Press.

Wainwright, J.L., Russell, S.T., and Patterson, C.J. (2004). Psychosocial adjustment school outcomes, and romantic relationships of adolescents with same-sex parents. Child Development, 75 (6), 1886-1898.

Wakschlag, L.S., Leventhal, B.L., Pine, D.S., Pickett, K.E. & Carter, A.S. (2006). Elucidating early mechanisms of developmental psychopathology: The case of parental smoking and disruptive behavior. Child Development, 77, 893-906.

Wang, Q. (2008). Emotion, knowledge, and autobiographical memory across the preschool years: A cross-cultural longitudinal investigation. Cognition, 108, 117-135.

Ward, K. (1994). Genetics and prenatal diagnosis. In J. R. Scott, P. J. DiSaia, C. B. Hammond, & W. N. Spellacy (Eds.), Dansforth's obstetrics and gynecology (7th ed.). Philadelphia: J. B. Lippincott.

Wechsler, D. (1975). Intelligence defined and undefined: A relativistic appraisal. American Psychologist, 30, 135-139.

Wentworth, N., Benson, J.B., & Haith, M.M. (2000). The development of infants' reaches for stationary and moving targets. Child Development, 71 (3), 576-601.

Westrin, A., and Lam, R.W. (2007). Seasonal affective disorder: A clinical update. Journal of Clinical Psychiatry, 29, 239-246.

Widiger, T.A., and Bornstein, R.F. (2001), Histrionic, dependent, and narcissistic personality disorders. In H.E. Adams and P.B.

Sutker (Eds.), Comprehensive handbook of psychopathology (pp. 509-534). New York: Kluwer Academic.

Zimmerman, A.W., Connors, S.L., & Pardo-Villamizar, C.A. (2006). Neuroimmunology and neurotransmitters in autism. In R. Tuchmen & I. Rapin (Eds.) Autism: A neurological disorder of early brain development (pp. 141-159). International Review of Child Neurology. London: Mac Keith Press.

Zimmermann, P., Maier, M.A., Winter, M., & Grossmann, K.E. (2001) Attachment and adolescents' emotion regulation during a joint problem-solving task with a friend. International Journal of Behavioral Development 25 (4), 331-343.